A Century of Caring

One Hundred Years of Organized
Veterinary Medicine in Ohio

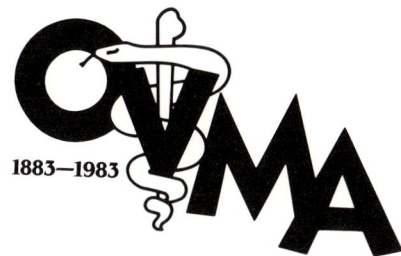

The Ohio Veterinary Medical Association
1883–1983

A Century of Caring
One Hundred Years of Organized Veterinary Medicine in Ohio

ISBN: 0-9613273-0-8

Published 1984 by the Ohio Veterinary Medical Association, Columbus
First Edition

Writing/research/editorial assistance:
Richard Compton

Project management:
Mark Luetke
Mark Tooman

Designers:
Jennifer Day
Robert Wilson

Production assistance:
Janis Lambert
Patricia Heckel

Copyrighted 1984 by the Ohio Veterinary Medical Association. Copyright under the Uniform Copyright Convention. All rights reserved. This book is protected by copyright. No part of it may be reproduced, stored in a retrieval system, or transmitted in any form or by any means, electronic, mechanical, photocopying, recording, or otherwise, without the written permission of the publisher. Made in the United States of America. Printed and distributed by Braun-Brumfield, Inc., Ann Arbor, Michigan 48106. Library of Congress catalog number 84-060216.

Dedicated to those many men and women—
past, present and future—
whose contributions have and will
continue to guide and shape the veterinary
profession in Ohio.

FOREWORD

The growth of professional veterinary medicine and the Ohio Veterinary Medical Association are the result of mutually cooperative efforts. So too is this history, which chronicles in words and pictures the major events of the past Century of Caring.

The OVMA is deeply indebted to the members of the Publication Committee—Drs. Milton Wyman, C. Roger Smith, Clyde Purdy, Thomas D. Young and James H. Rosenberger—for the time and talent they generously committed to this Centennial project. Its successful completion is due, in large measure, to their dedicated work.

Other OVMA members also made important contributions. The association is grateful to Drs. Clinton D. Barrett, George T. Bear, Harry Goldstein, John W. Jackman, Philip W. Murdick, Arch C. Priestly and Vernon L. Tharp for the counsel, historic material and personal recollections they provided during the preparation of this history. Special thanks also are due and warmly conveyed to the OVMA staff, Gene King, Barbara Madison, and Debbie Conklin, for so willingly assuming the additional responsibilities connected with this ambitious project. As always, the staff's commitment and efforts were outstanding.

Particular recognition should go to Richard Compton for his comprehensive writing, research and editorial assistance in preparing the manuscript and selecting photos for the book. Also important was the role of the firm of Flournoy and Gibbs in establishing the tone and overall direction of this project and assuring its completion—especially Mark Luetke and Mark Tooman, project coordination; Jennifer Day and Robert Wilson, design; and Janis Lambert and Patricia Heckel, production assistance.

In addition, the OVMA deeply appreciates the research assistance provided by Ruth Jones, OSU Photo Archives; Arlene Peterson, Ohio Historical Society; and Roberta Garrett, OSU College of Veterinary Medicine Library.

The results of this cooperative venture are recorded on the succeeding pages. It is your Century of Caring—read and enjoy.

THE OHIO VETERINARY
MEDICAL ASSOCIATION

CONTENTS

Prologue ix
The Historic Perspective.............. 1
The Birth of the OVMA 13
The Growth of Education 27
Animal Disease:
The Great Campaign................ 43
The '20s and '30s:
New Concerns & Opportunities 55
Post War:
Expansion and New Directions....... 71
OSU:
The Later Years 81
Veterinary Medicine:
The Military Connection 97
The OVMA Auxiliary 101
Epilogue:
The Future...................... 107
Past OVMA and
Auxiliary Presidents................ 108
Bibliography..................... 109
Index 111

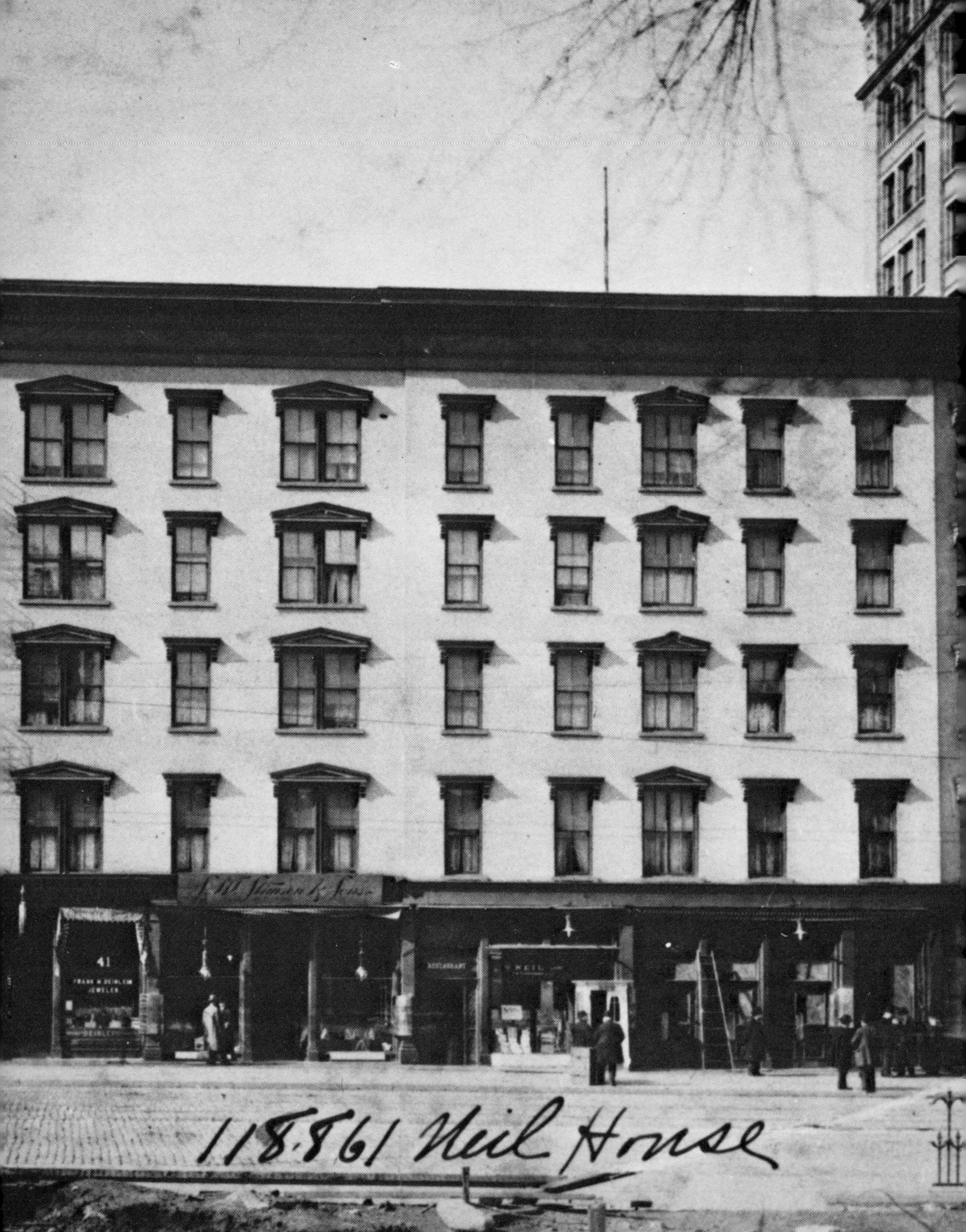

OVMA History
PROLOGUE

The date: July 24, 1883. Headlines in the *Columbus Dispatch* of that day revealed a growing concern over threats to public health. New Orleans was preparing to take precautionary measures against the spread of yellow fever from the Caribbean area and both Europe and the United States were nervously watching the devastating progress of a cholera epidemic in Egypt that was killing hundreds every day. Health officials in Washington were calling for the strictest quarantine measures to keep both diseases out of the country.

Other front page stories included a report on the continuing Western Union strike, a dispatch from Baltimore, Maryland, on the collapse of a resort pier that claimed 60 to 70 lives, and a brief report about a small tornado that had taken the roof off a warehouse in Newcomerstown, Ohio.

All of this was front page news on July 24. There was also another story, much closer to home, but it developed too late for the *Dispatch* deadline and it was not until the following day, July 25, that the paper took note of it in a brief summary on one of the inner pages:

> After discussing various topics in regard to elevating the standard of the profession, the veterinary surgeons effected a permanent organization yesterday afternoon and elected officers for the ensuing year as follows: President, W.C. Fair, Cleveland; First Vice President, J.V. Newton, Toledo; Second Vice President, T.B. Cotton, Mt. Vernon; Third Vice President, A. Moor, Mansfield; Secretary, J.M. Waddel, Columbus; Corresponding Secretary, J.S. Butler, Piqua; Treasurer, T.B. Hillock, Columbus; Board of Censors, T.G. Marlin, Urbana; L.B. Chase, Berlin; and W.F. Derr, Mansfield. T.E. Daniels of Chicago, and Professor Townshend of this city were elected honorary members. The meeting then adjourned to meet at the Fairgrounds, this city, on the 5th of September.

This July 24 meeting, so succinctly noted by the *Dispatch,* did not at the time rank in editorial importance with a Mideast cholera epidemic, a Maryland pier collapse, or even an errant Ohio tornado. But succeeding years would confirm it as one of the most significant events of the day, to be remembered long after the front page headlines were forgotten. Because it marked the founding of The Ohio State Veterinary Medical Association, now the Ohio Veterinary Medical Association (OVMA).

Still, the *Columbus Dispatch* really can't be faulted for relegating the story to a few lines on an inner page. In 1883, the initial effort of a handful of Ohio veterinary surgeons to elevate their profession had little claim on public attention. Indeed, in the minds of many people, veterinary medicine wasn't a profession at all; it was the necessary avocation of farmers and livestock men and the self-taught, unscientific vocation of "hoss doctors" and "cow-leeches," the latter coming from the ranks of blacksmiths, grooms, teamsters and other animal handlers who parlayed their limited knowledge into roles as rural medicine men. The professionally-trained veterinarian was an exception; in the United States during the second half of the 1800s, it was estimated there were 500 poorly-trained practitioners for every well-trained veterinarian. Small wonder that the veterinarian was not a figure of considerable public prominence.

It was this situation that troubled the founders of the Ohio Veterinary Medical Association and brought them together. This book is the story of what they and their successors achieved during "A Century of Caring."

OSVMA/OVMA

When our Association was founded in 1883, it was known as the Ohio State *Veterinary Medical Association (OSVMA). "State" was not dropped from the title until 1965 when it became the Ohio Veterinary Medical Association (OVMA). However, for consistency, OVMA is used throughout this book* except *when the original title is part of a quote from historic records.*

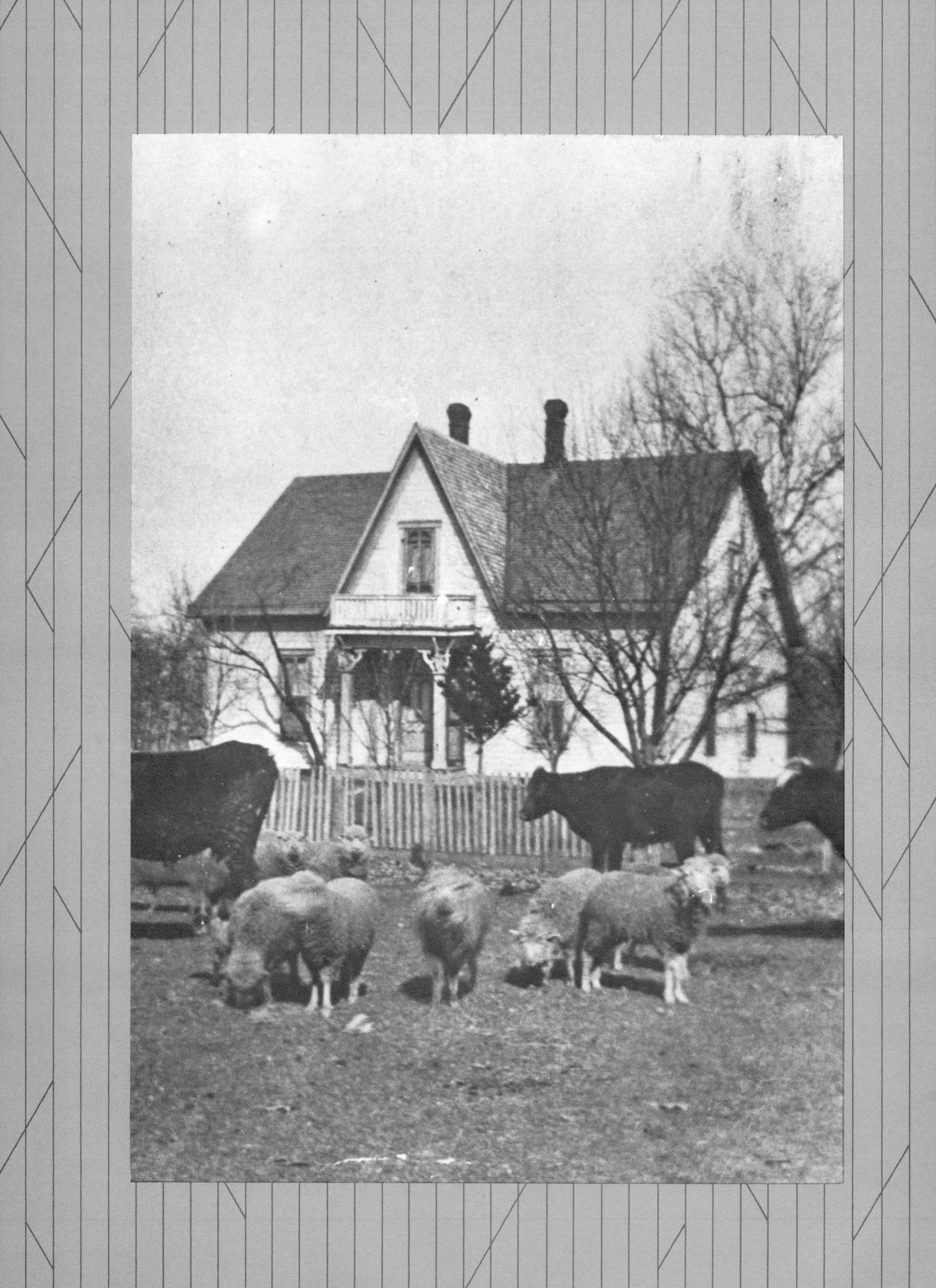

CHAPTER I

THE HISTORIC PERSPECTIVE

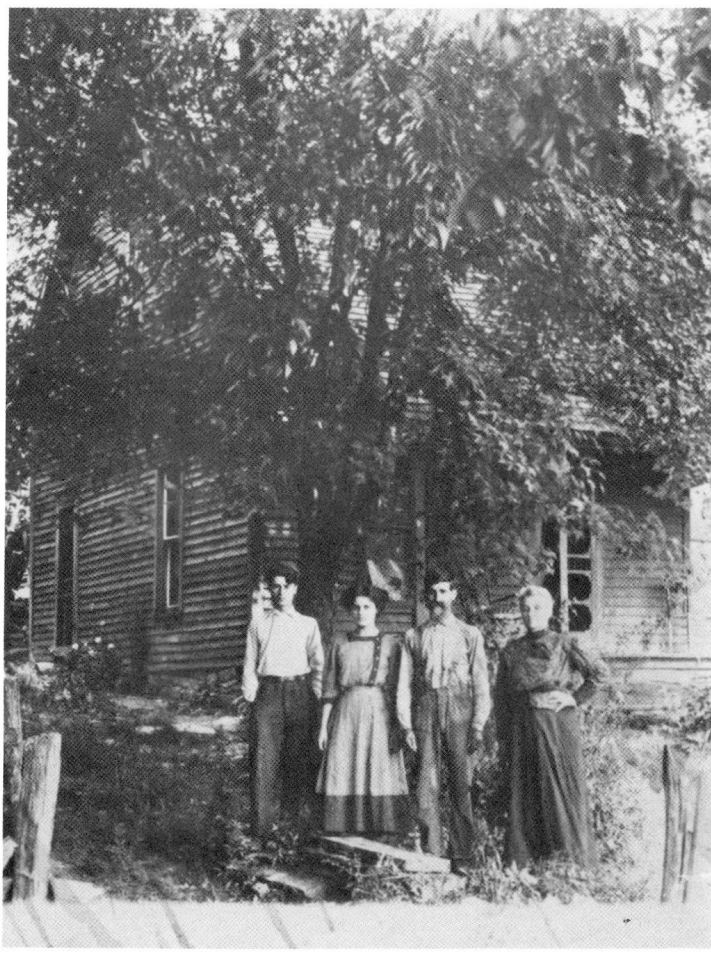

Rural Ohio was not as peaceful and trouble-free as these turn-of-the-century pictures suggest. Farmers still had to cope with recurring outbreaks of disease that often reached epidemic proportions and destroyed hundreds of thousands of animals. (Ohio Historical Society)

There still exists a bucolic image of rural Ohio (and all of rural America) in the late 1800s: sturdy horses, sleek cattle, fat hogs, and thick-wooled sheep. Placid and pastoral, it seems, in retrospect, a trouble-free world still resisting the noxious invasion of the industrial revolutionaries.

But the image, inviting as it is, does not hold up under close scrutiny. Rural, Ohio may have been; trouble-free, it was not. With over 26,000 acres of farmland, valued at close to three-quarters of a billion dollars, and hundreds of thousands of head of valuable livestock, Ohio, like the rest of rural America, was beset with problems. And one of the most pressing was animal disease of epidemic proportions.

Hog cholera, which was first identified in Ohio in 1833, decimated herds and ruined farmers. In one six-year period prior to 1885, close to 900,000 Ohio hogs died from the disease.

Nationally, during the 1870s, hog cholera was responsible for 90 percent of swine mortality at a cost of more than $20,000,000 a year; in a single year, 1885, the disease killed 2,000,000 hogs in Iowa. It was a farm nightmare from which there seemed to be no awakening; reporting on an outbreak in the Cincinnati area in 1857, *The American Veterinary Journal* noted: "The disease is considered incurable, having baffled the most critical investigation into its nature, and has steadily resisted all remedial agents."

And hog cholera was only one plague on the rural house. Other infectious diseases were also increasingly prevalent: glanders of horses, tuberculosis of cattle, pleuropneumonia, Texas Fever, and foot rot in sheep. Regardless of his choice of livestock, the Ohio farmer, and his counterparts across the nation, lived with the ever-present fear of some devastating affliction that would consume animal life and income.

There were a number of reasons for the disease problem. In many states, farm animals roamed loose and maladies were easily spread. Many farmers also compelled their animals to forage outside all winter, a practice that made them more susceptible to disease. And, most pernicious, was the total absence of regulations governing importation or interstate shipment of livestock. Diseased animals could be brought into the country or moved through it at will and avaricious livestock "hustlers" took advantage of the situation, all the while stubbornly resisting efforts to impose controls. To the latter group goes the dubious distinction of having made a major contribution to the spread of livestock disease.

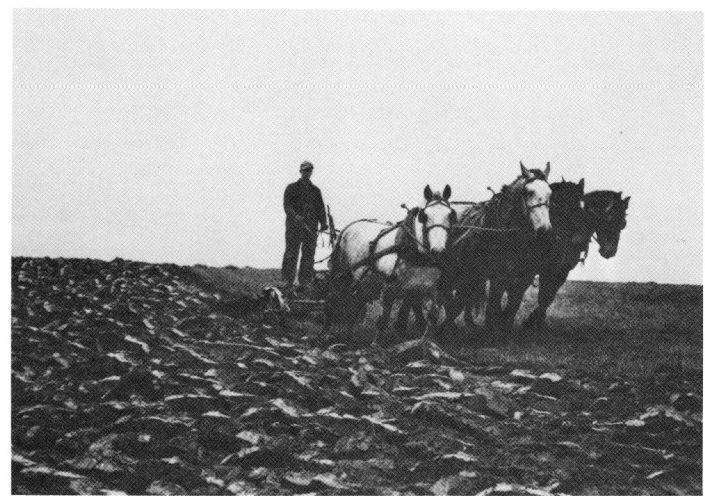

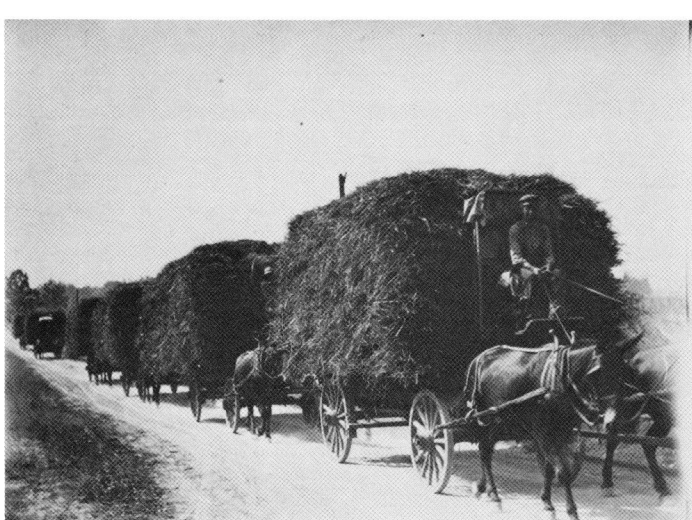

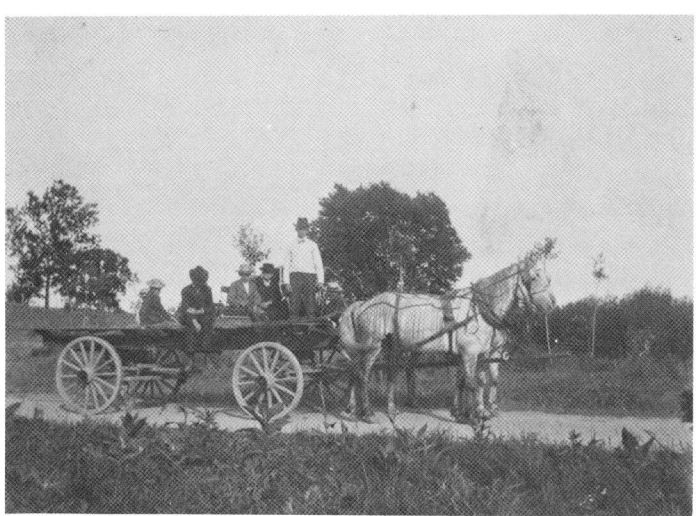

Horses and mules remained kings of the road and field well into the 20th Century. Both trained veterinarians and untrained "animal doctors" emphasized equine care since farmers were dependent on their draft animals for transportation and field labor. (Ohio Historical Society)

But costly as these destructive practices may have been, they were not the only causes of animal death on an epizootic scale. The lack of professional animal care was also a factor; in the late 1800s, American agriculture was paying the price for a short-sighted neglect of scientific veterinary medicine that had persisted for nearly three-quarters of a century. The professional veterinarian, who could have been a front-line defense against disease, was restricted by numbers alone at this point to little more than guerrilla action. It was a situation that led to the caustic observation, recorded by Earl W. Hayter in

> *The Troubled Farmer,* that "no country in the world had as many animals or took less interest in their behalf" than the United States.

Ohio was no exception to this observation. In his history of the OSU College of Veterinary Medicine, Professor Arthur F. Schalk notes:

> The history of veterinary medicine in the State of Ohio, to the time of the founding of the Ohio Agricultural and Mechanical College (OSU) in 1870, did not differ materially from that which existed throughout the nation during those years.... Suffice to state that during that period of nearly 70 years, there was virtually no scientific veterinary education in the state. Consequently, all animal diseases were left to the mercy of the laity.

The laity is divided by Professor Schalk into "two rather distinct groups" and of the first he writes:

> A good number of so-called, self-designated Doctors of Animals... not infrequently these imposters not only were wholly ignorant as regards the healing arts, but entirely wanting in knowledge of even the most rudimentary principles of livestock care and management. The operations of a large majority of them rarely attained the level of mediocrity. It is now history that often great losses in livestock followed in the wake of their activities.

Considering the treatments administered by many of these "Doctors of Animals," the losses are understandable and Professor Schalk's use of the word "mercy" takes on a note of irony. In large measure, their activities seemed to encompass what might be called the three "B's" of barbaric treatment: bleeding, blistering, and burning. In his book *The Troubled Farmer,* Earl W. Hayter writes that "horses were often bled until they could hardly stand. Whatever the animal's condition or disease, the quack usually decided it needed bleeding because it was an easy operation that produced a fee."

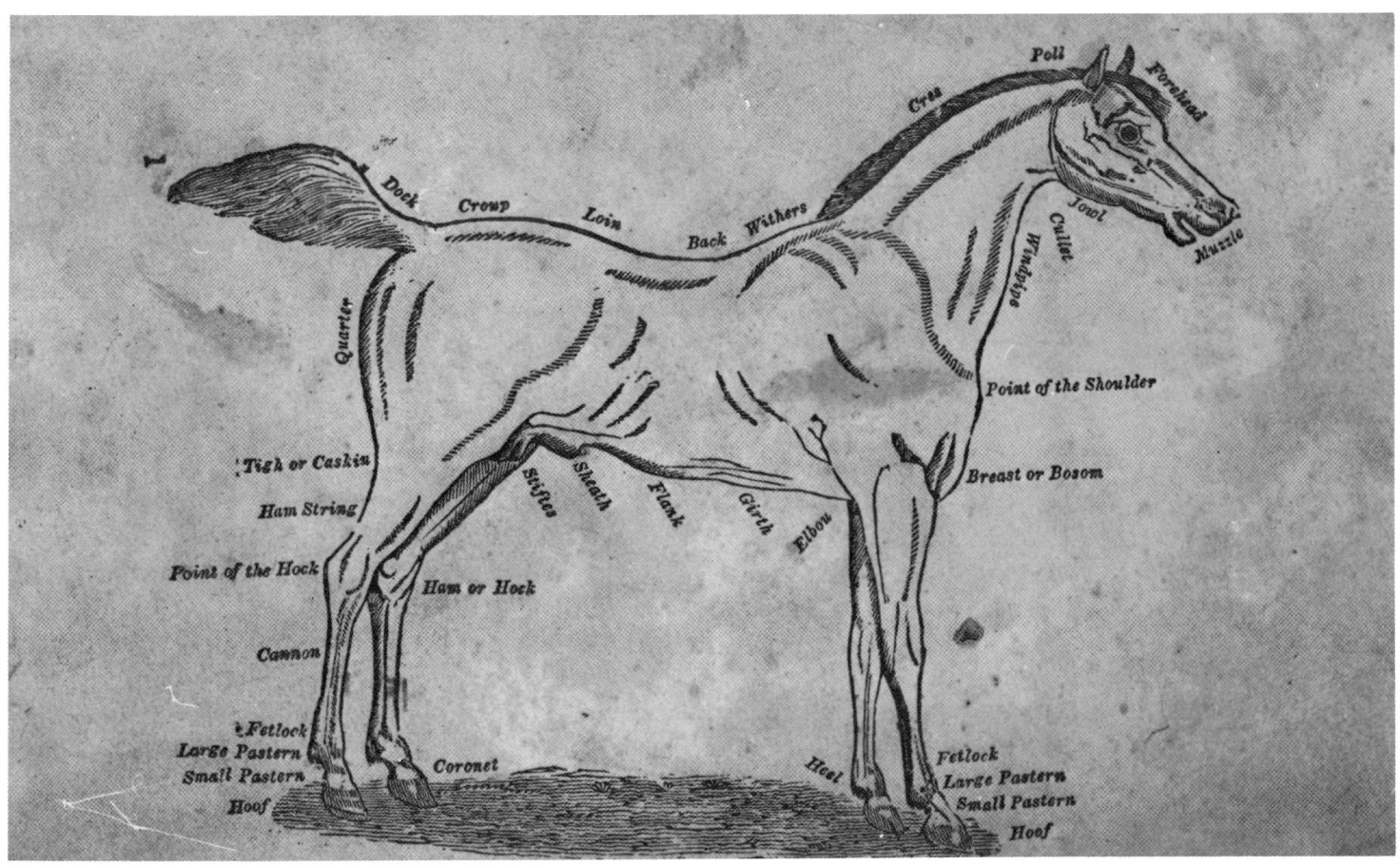
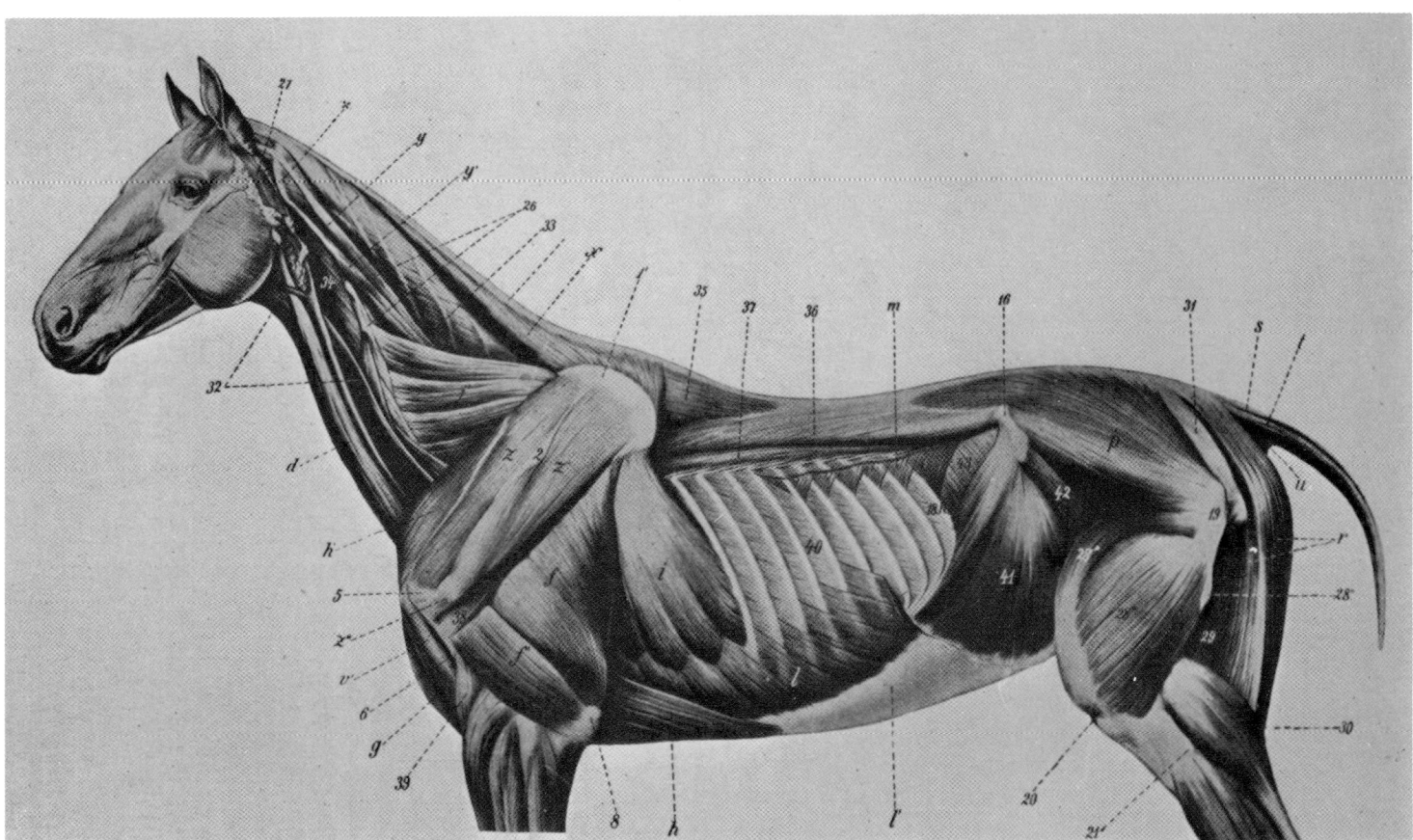

The contrast between these pictures is dramatic evidence of the progress of veterinary medicine. The superficial sketch is from The United States Farriery, *published in 1853; the detailed anatomical illustration is from the 1914 edition of Dr. Septimus Sisson's comprehensive* The Anatomy of Domestic Animals. *(Ohio Historical Society)*

Hayter also noted that self-styled "medicine men" treated lampas, a congestion of a horse's mucuous membrane that sometimes interfered temporarily with eating habits, by burning the roof of the animal's mouth with a red-hot poker. And of other treatments, he writes: "Quacks also used strong purgatives and drenches in often enormous quantities. Favorite contents included dragon's blood, black antimony, sulphur, spices, sometimes the animal's own excretions. In some parts of the country strong mineral poisons, acids and preparations of arsenic, antimony and mercury were also used."

There were many other barbaric treatments designed to cure a host of often imaginary afflictions; a complete listing would create the distinct impression that in this period an animal's greatest enemy was not disease, but the men who came to treat it. (And the men often were.) But this would be an unbalanced interpretation of history. The "quacks" and "medicine men" who took advantage of the neglect of professional veterinary medicine were not the only untrained practitioners; there were others, well-meaning and not entirely unskilled, who coped with the results of that neglect and did the best they could. They comprised the second group of laity and of them Professor Schalk writes:

> Another group was composed largely of herdsmen, shepherds, general caretakers and stock owners. Usually they were men of sound judgment who had obtained considerable practical knowledge of animal husbandry in the daily care and management of their herds and flocks ... these men resorted mostly to preventive measures in handling the ills of their animals ... they did not profess medical knowledge ... they did some ministering chiefly with home remedies ... this combined with good hygiene and self-inflicted quarantines materially lessened losses and curbed the spread of transmissible diseases. Those practices, while they may not fully comply with the best professional principles of today, served a good purpose. ...

So the picture of animal care in the mid and late 1800s was not entirely bleak. Some efforts were being made to deal with animal diseases on a rational basis, with practices incorporating observation and experience. But these efforts, though well-intentioned and sometimes productive, were still largely unscientific and unsuccessful; they were not an effective response to the plagues which periodically swept Ohio and the rest of the nation.

The people who could have responded effectively were not there, at least not in any significant number. In 1847, there were only 15 graduate veterinarians in the United States; in 1850, there were 46. From this point on there was a steady increase, but no relationship between numbers and need. In 1880, the United States, with 131,000,000 head of livestock, had only 2,130 graduate veterinarians. And many of these were from European schools, where scientific veterinary medicine had its roots.

The history of veterinary medicine is as lengthy as the history of civilized man. From the days when animals were first domesticated (as early as 8,000 B.C.), people have been concerned about their health, and it seems safe to assume that even the earliest herdsmen applied what primitive treatment they could to ailing livestock. Their efforts (and results) are lost forever, but archaeologists and historians probing the less distant past have found records that indicate a very active interest in animal health and the treatment of disease.

Babylon's Code of Hammurabi, promulgated around 2200 B.C., included veterinary writings and Egypt produced the Veterinary Papyrus of Kahun about 1900 B.C. In the same period, India had a distinct veterinary profession and has given us the first

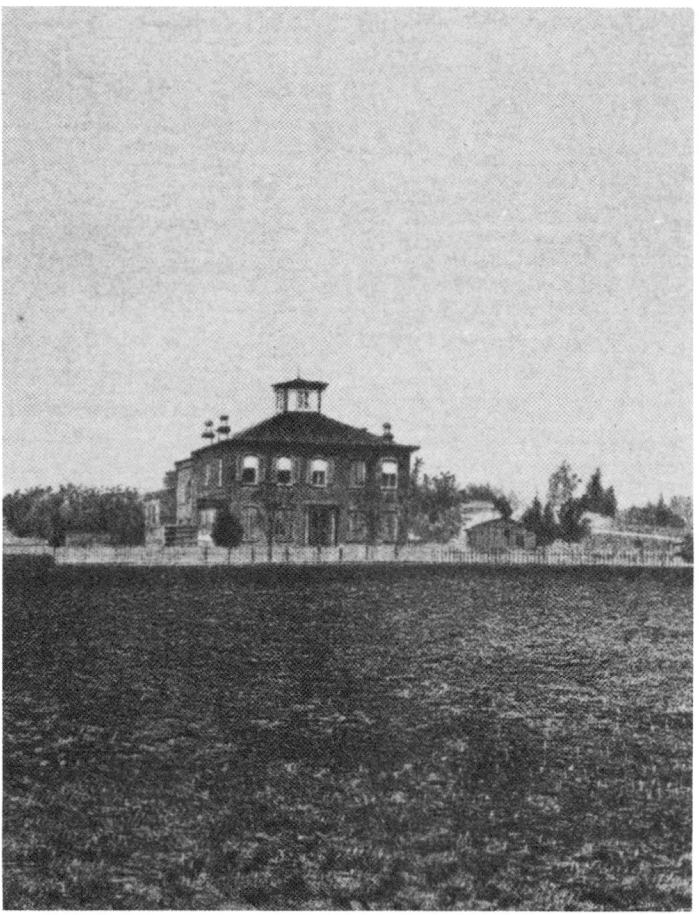

The Bureau of Animal Industry Veterinary Station at the U.S. Department of Agriculture, Washington, D.C., 1884. Establishment of the BAI in 1884 was the first major action taken by the federal government to deal with the critical problem of animal plagues and epizootics. (Ohio Historical Society)

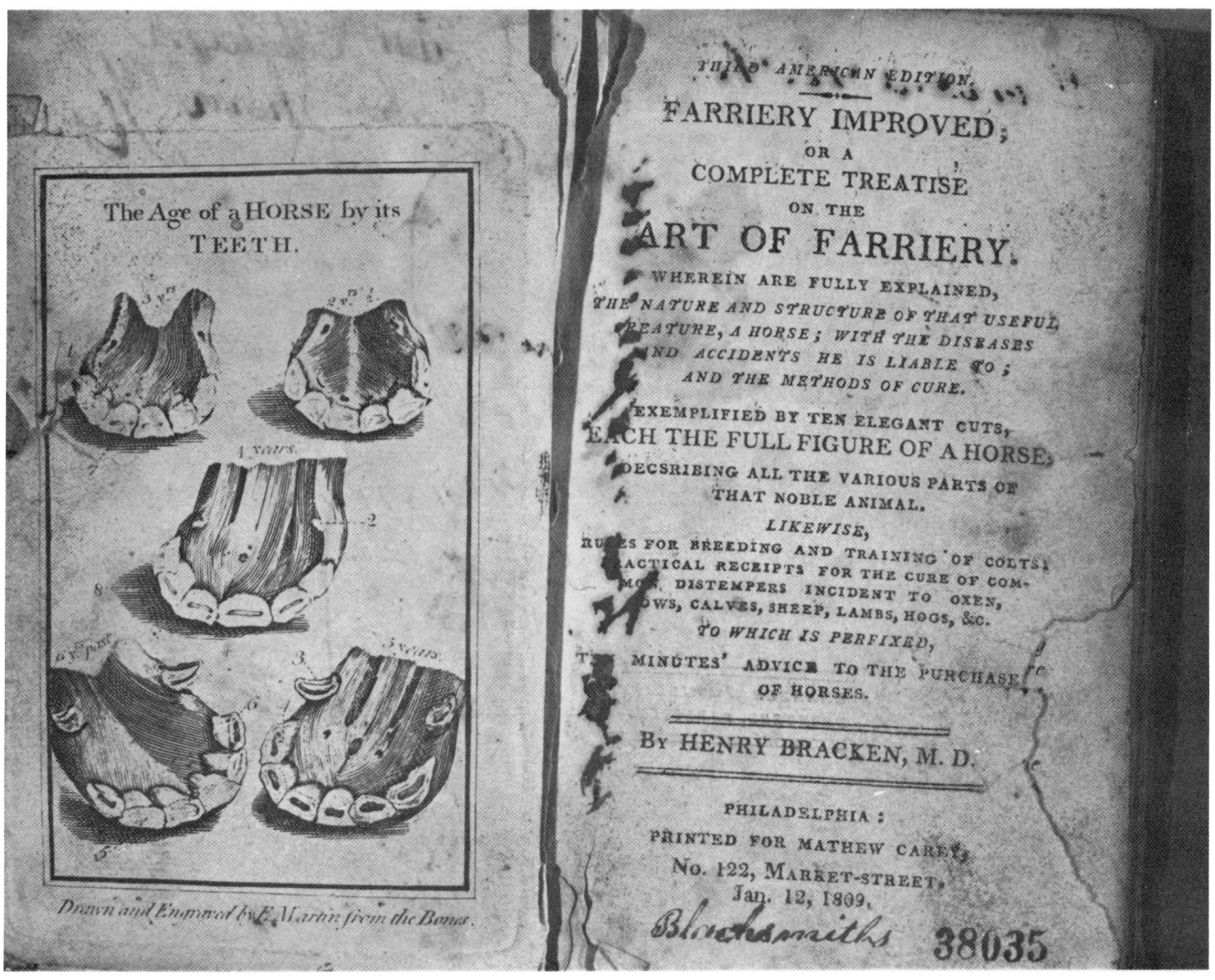

One of the earliest books on animal care printed in the United States, the Art of Farriery, *was published in Philadelphia in 1809. Note that the author is an M.D.; at this time the graduate veterinarian was virtually nonexistent in America. (Ohio Historical Society)*

recorded listing of a veterinarian's name; he was Salihotra, who lived about 1800 B.C.

Later records include fragments of an old book on veterinary science with prescriptions for the treatment of ailing horses; it was excavated in Syria in 1939. Compiled by the Captain of the Household Cavalry of the King of Ugarit (about 1400 B.C.) it included this recommended treatment:

> If a horse has a sore nose, prepare a salve from figs and raisins, mixed with oatmeal and liquid. This liquid should be poured into the horse's nostrils.

In Greek and Roman times, veterinary medicine became more sophisticated, having drawn the attention of some of the period's most advanced philosophers and medical writers. Dr. W.W. Armistead, writing on *The Ascent of Veterinary Medical Education* in the *Journal of the AVMA*, notes that men like Hippocrates and Aristotle dealt with the diseases of both animals and people, adding that "Aristotle's observations on the incidence and treatment of animal diseases were astonishingly accurate—often more so than were the observations on astronomy for which he is better known."

Also accurate was the Greek physician Galen (130–201 A.D.), who brought to veterinary medicine an insight that, unfortunately, would not be heeded for centuries to come. Dr. Arthur Schalk cites him as "the first writer to acknowledge one medicine for all animal kind, including man . . . he recognized that the human family was susceptible to many animal diseases and championed the idea that all food animals should be inspected and pronounced safe and wholesome before being used for human consumption."

Some three centuries after Galen, a Roman, Vegetius Renatus (450-500 A.D.) compiled the first book

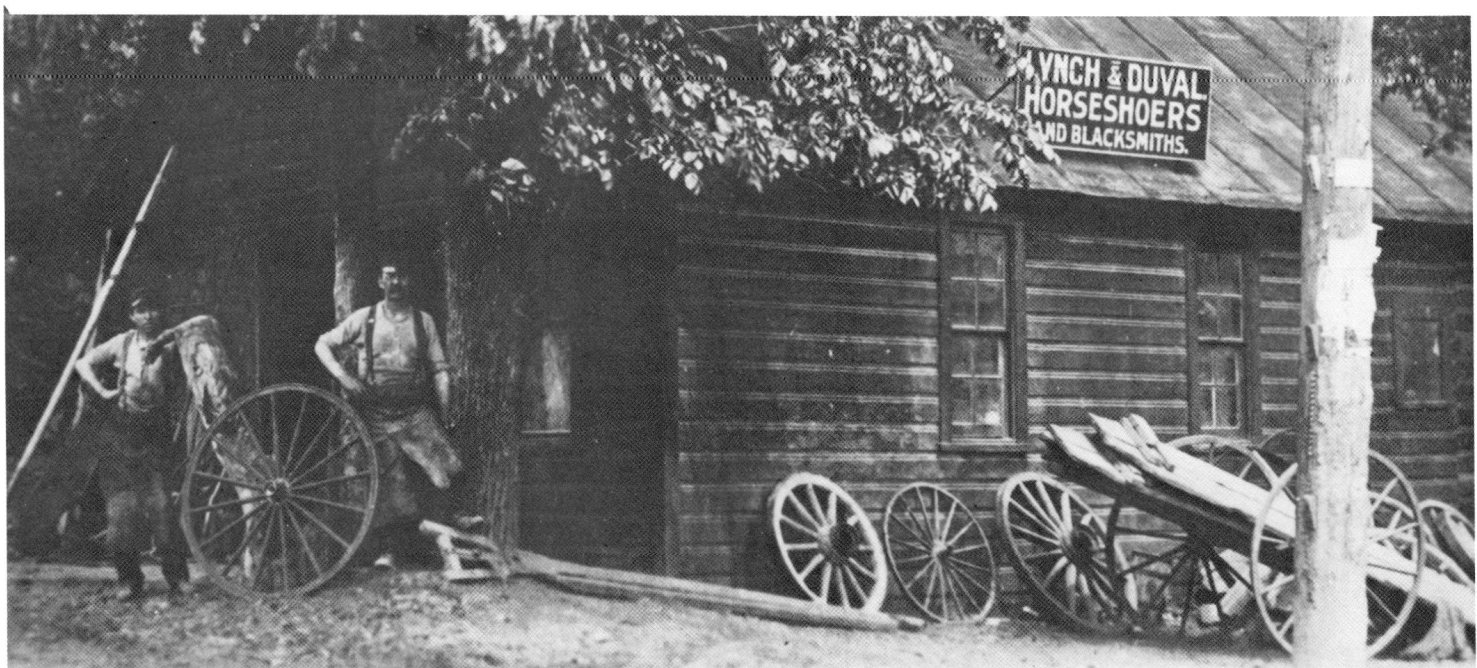

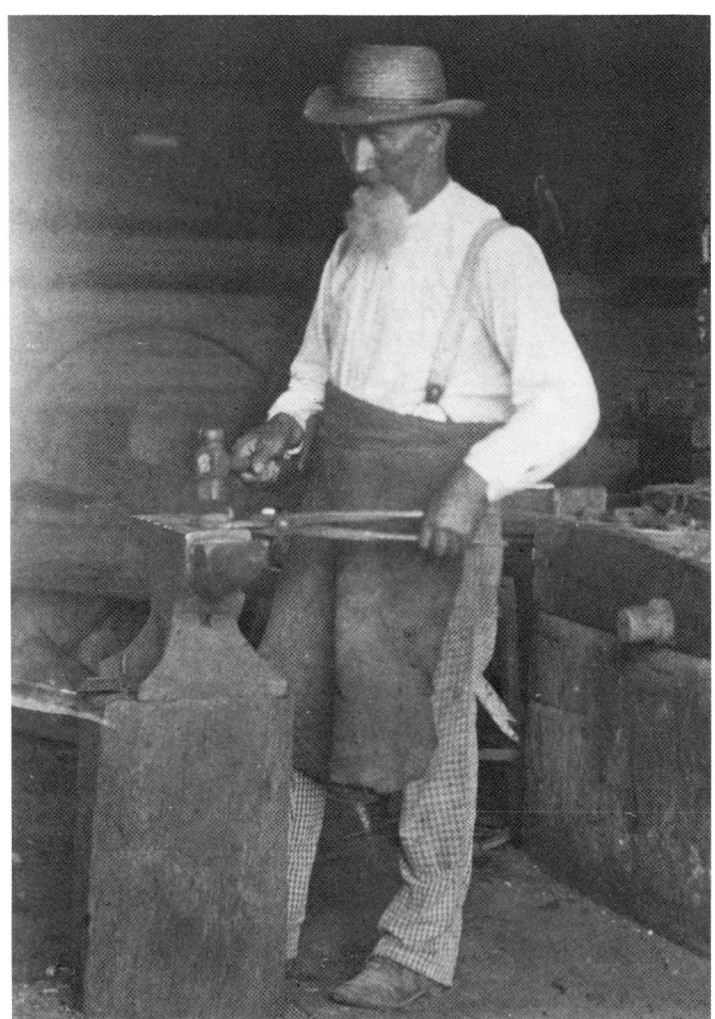

In the absence of trained veterinarians, many blacksmiths and other animal handlers doubled as untrained "hoss doctors." A few were well-intentioned and reasonably competent, but most had little knowledge of animal care and their often barbaric treatments did more harm than good. (Ohio Historical Society)

of the Christian era devoted entirely to veterinary medicine. Like his illustrious predecessors, he did much to advance the profession and of him, Dr. Schalk has written:

> In the annals of veterinary medicine there are no sounder medical philosophies and doctrines than those found in the writings of Vegetius.... Vegetius merits the distinction of being called the father of veterinary medicine.

The achievements of these early philosophers and medical writers conferred on veterinary medicine a portion of "the glory that was Greece and the grandeur that was Rome." But the honor was transitory and the progress short-lived. Because, with the collapse of the Roman Empire, veterinary medicine, like the other arts and sciences, fell victim to the suffocating environment of the Dark Ages. Whatever forward momentum the profession had attained was lost over the long centuries of Europe's intellectual midnight and what had been a province of Aristotle became the property of illiterate medieval blacksmiths.

The blacksmiths (farriers) owned veterinary practice for a long time and might have held it even longer, but for the intervention of calamity. This time it was not imperial collapse; it was invasion by a disease called rinderpest.

Between 1711 and 1769 this plague killed over 200,000,000 cattle in western Europe; in just four years, 1710–14, it wiped out one-half of the cattle in France. It was an epizootic catastrophe and blacksmiths were of no help at all. Europe needed trained veterinarians and anxious governments set out to rediscover what men like Galen and Vegetius had been talking about centuries before.

France was the first to act. The Council of State established the world's first modern veterinary school at Lyon in 1762 and a second school at Alfort in 1766. Other European countries were soon to follow: Austria in 1767; Denmark, 1773; Germany, 1774 and 1787; Italy, 1769, 1776, and 1790; Poland, 1784; Hungary, 1787; and England, 1793.

The schools produced results. At Lyon, veterinarian Peter Camper determined that rinderpest arose from natural causes, scoring a beat on human medical researchers who were also addressing the problem. By the end of the 18th century, French veterinarians were also focusing on the role of infectious agents in a host of diseases and developing methods for controlling them. Similar advances were being made at other European schools.

The long night of scientific veterinary medicine was finally over. But while the sun was beginning to shine in Europe, it would be several decades before it pierced the clouds over the United States.

Historians cite several reasons for the painfully slow development of professional veterinary medicine in America. One obstacle was created by the traditional ties between the United States and England; as a result the U.S. was to a great extent dependent on British veterinary leadership and that leadership lagged well behind the Continent in veterinary science.

Another was the attitude of the U.S. government, which stood in sharp contrast to that of European governments. For years, despite rampant epidemics, the U.S. Department of Agriculture did little to encourage the development of the veterinary profession.

A third obstacle was the attitude of many American farmers. They were often slow to accept trained veterinarians, seeing them as one more manifestation of the urban society, industry and science which they mistrusted. Writing in *The Troubled Farmer*, Earl W. Hayter observed that:

> They tended to cling . . . to traditional ways, to continue to give their loyalties to the old ideals and values of the agrarian society. Their faith in the old remedies transcended their faith in scientific ones.

This attitude also led farmers to resist efforts to control quacks and nonprofessionals. And here it was more than a case of clinging to traditional ways; the farmers had a very practical objection, too. Again quoting Hayter:

> . . . farmers contended that if laws were passed giving the right to practice to trained veterinarians alone, a large percentage of the nonprofessional practitioners would be barred from performing their services, a situation that would create a serious problem in areas miles removed from the nearest professionals.

Considering that as late as 1890 most localities lacked a trained veterinarian, the farmer's concern was a real one. But the problem, in part, was of their

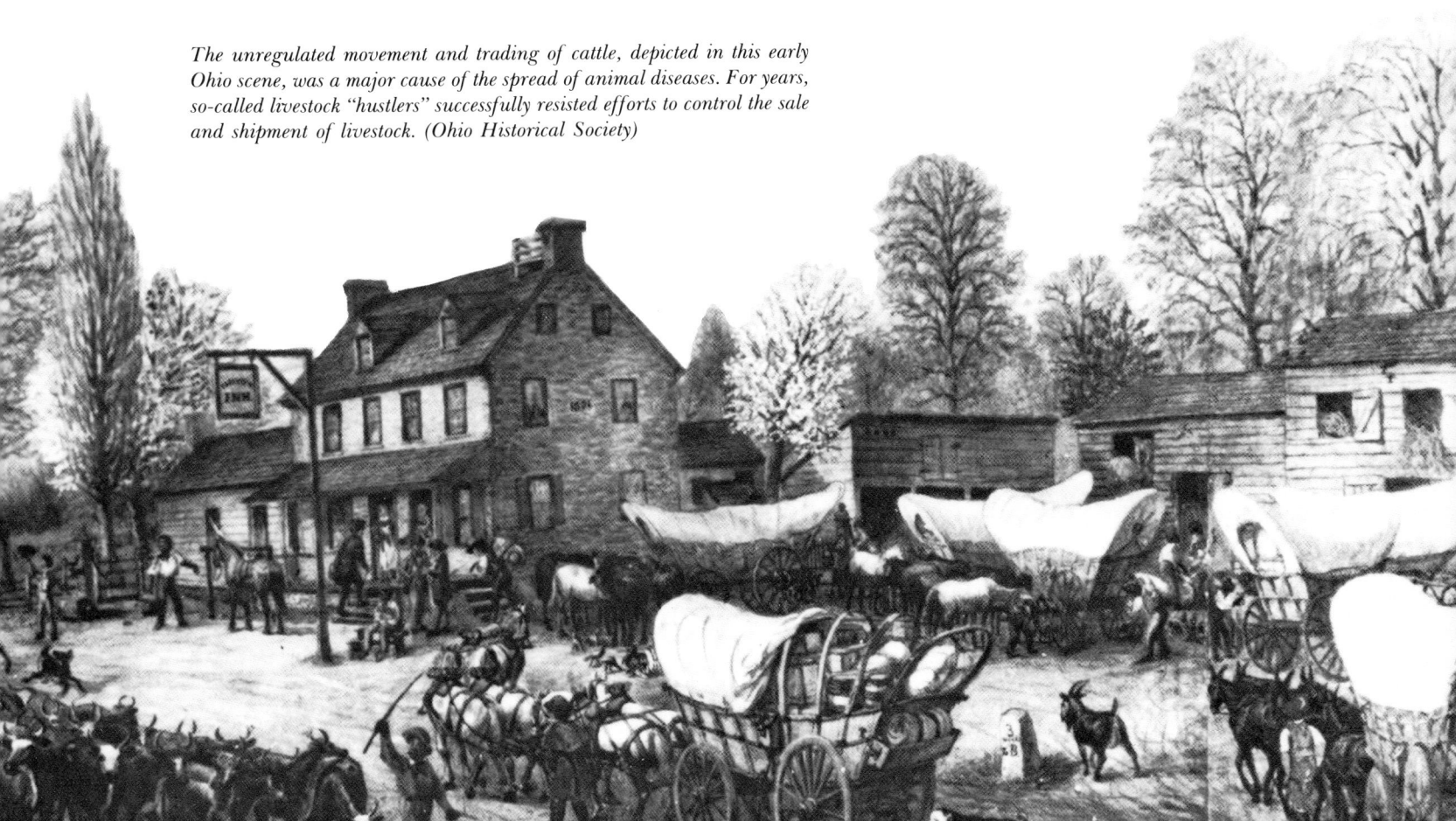

The unregulated movement and trading of cattle, depicted in this early Ohio scene, was a major cause of the spread of animal diseases. For years, so-called livestock "hustlers" successfully resisted efforts to control the sale and shipment of livestock. (Ohio Historical Society)

THE
UNITED STATES FARRIERY

AND

ZOOLOGICAL HISTORY

OF

HORSES, CATTLE, SHEEP, HOGS, AND BEES;

CONNECTED WITH THE

THERAPEUTICAL ILLUSTRATIONS OF MEDICINE.

"MULTUM IN PARVO."

WITH ENGRAVINGS.

COMPILED FROM THE MOST APPROVED AUTHORS, BY
BUELL EASTMAN, M. D.,
AUTHOR OF A NEW "MEDICAL PRACTICE AND TREATISE ON HUMAN DISEASES."

SECOND EDITION, REVISED AND ENLARGED.

CINCINNATI:
PUBLISHED BY C. CROPPER & SON.
1853.

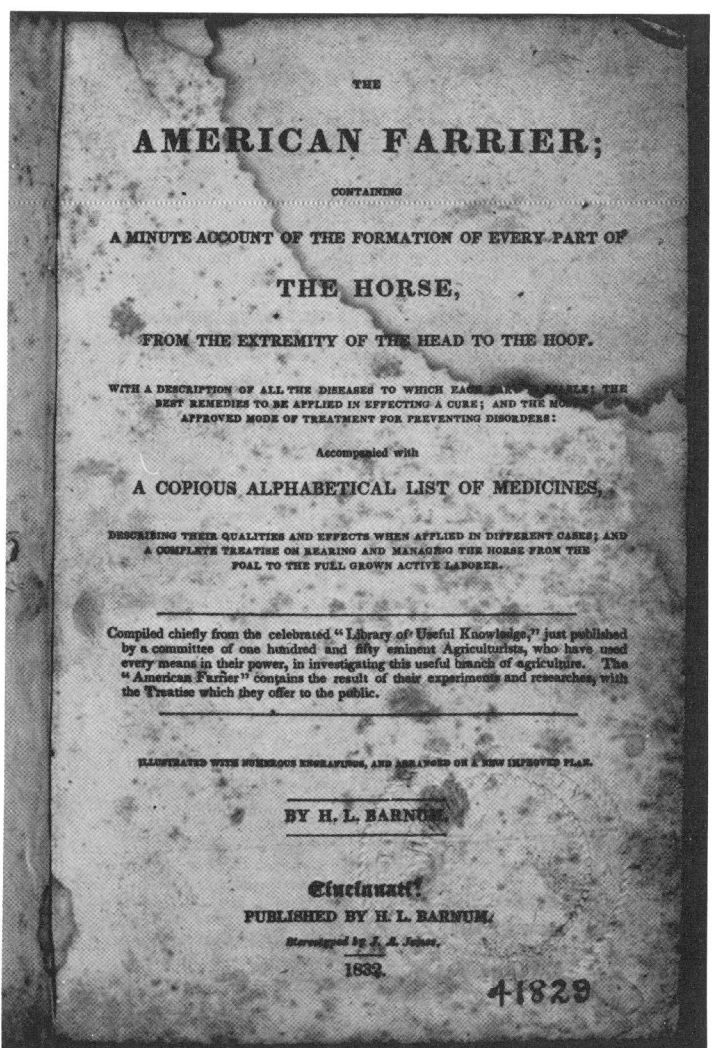

Two Ohio texts on farriery from 1832 and 1853, both published in Cincinnati. Books like these were a major source of animal care information throughout much of the 19th Century. Some were valuable, others not worth the paper they were printed on. (Ohio Historical Society)

own making since farm attitudes were a factor in limiting the number of professionals.

Obviously, the most destructive effect of these obstacles was that they seriously impeded the progress of veterinary education. In the face of government neglect and rural suspicion, it was difficult to generate strong interest in the creation of veterinary schools. The result was that more than a century after Europe awoke to the need for scientific veterinary training, the United States was still, by comparison, an educational wasteland. Figures cited by Hayter make the point:

In 1877, Prussia with one-third as many animals as the U.S., had as many as five veterinary colleges maintained by the state. France had three superior veterinary schools. Great Britain, with only about one-half our livestock, had four colleges. But the U.S., with two to three times as many animals as any of these countries, had not a single college of national importance, and none that was maintained by public funds. There were two or three struggling private colleges in the East... most western states had no veterinary schools of any kind.

The point in time, 1877, is worth noting. It was only six years before the founding of the Ohio Veterinary Medical Association.

But if the mills of American veterinary medicine ground slowly during much of the 19th century, they were at least moving. There was no ground-swell of public support for veterinary education, but throughout the period far-sighted individuals and organizations pressed for the establishment of veterinary schools. Agricultural societies, individual farm leaders, the agricultural press, and the nation's small advance guard of professional veterinarians wore away at public indifference and gradually shaped a beginning for American veterinary medicine.

Their efforts were not always successful; indeed it would be the last quarter of the century before many of the early dreams began to be realized. The 1850s, for example, saw the establishment of the United States' first veterinary schools, The Veterinary College of Philadelphia in 1852 and the Boston Veterinary Institute in 1854. But both were false starts; there is no record of either school having turned out a graduate.

The same decade, however, saw the founding of America's first successful veterinary school, The New York College of Veterinary Surgeons, born in 1857. The college remained in operation for over forty years, graduating 291 veterinarians before closing its doors in 1899. It was the first of many private schools that came into existence during the last half of the 19th century.

Some of these schools were very bad; they offered little in the way of professional training and frequently supplemented their income by selling bogus diplomas by mail for $100 (or $135 if the diploma was adorned with the forged signature of a foreign scholar). But there were other private schools, like The New York College, which did a good job of educating veterinarians and their contributions were particularly important given the almost total absence of public-supported veterinary education.

Six years after the establishment of The New York College of Veterinary Surgeons there was another milestone, the founding in 1863 of the United States Veterinary Medical Association, now the American Veterinary Medical Association (AVMA). Formed to promote quality veterinary services, humane treatment, and self-improvement through education, the Association would in succeeding years become a powerful advocate of the professional veterinarian and scientific veterinary education. An Ohioan was among the Association's "Founding Forty"; he was Doctor George W. Bowler, of Cincinnati, who was elected a vice president at the group's first meeting in New York. Bowler would later become a charter member of the Ohio Veterinary Medical Association.

In this same period, the government was also becoming involved, although by an action not directly promoting veterinary medicine. Less than a year before the founding of USVMA, on July 2, 1862, Congress passed the Morrill Act, the federal land grant legislation that began "the democratization of higher education" by spurring the development of land grant colleges and universities across the United States. Since agricultural education would be a major concern of these institutions, it was an act that inevitably gave great impetus to veterinary medicine as a science and profession.

So progress was being made. And, equally important as the century progressed, public attitudes were beginning to change.

With animal diseases still rampant, the practices of folk medicine and itinerant "healers" were targets of increasing criticism. Focusing on the latter, one agricultural journal of the period observed:

> They work on the 'guess' system and treat all cases nearly alike; so that, if perchance an animal recovers under their treatment, it is in spite of it, and a case of pure luckiness, rather than the consequence of their skill.

And another journal took to task pseudo-veterinarians and their written efforts, complaining that:

> Every rural neighborhood is infested with the inevitable book agent who, with oily tongue, gulls the unsophisticated into purchasing some great Illustrated Stock Book or Illustrated Horse Doctor or Complete Farrier, some other catchpenny, swindling affair, not worth the white paper it is printed upon.

More and more, people were questioning the "old ways" of animal care and those who practiced them. There was, of course, no abrupt turning away from the past; the records show that quacks and self-appointed medicine men continued to flourish for years to come. But now, for the first time, their dominance was being challenged. Scientific veterinary medicine was finally emerging from the shadows, drawn out by a growing recognition of its importance.

(A parenthetical note seems justified here to put in perspective the acceptance of "quackery" in the treatment of animal disease. The same willingness to accept spurious "doctoring" was just as evident in matters of human health. Ads and correspondence in *The Ohio Farmer* of the period included recommendations for cancer cures, among them a "best ever" salve made from red oak bark and dogwood roots, and the inspired testimonial of a man who said he owed his life to "Warners Safe Cure" and felt duty-bound to "make an open declaration . . . for the benefit of suffering humanity." The last quarter of the 19th century was also a golden age of human medical quackery.)

The progress of veterinary medicine in the last quarter of the 1800s was the result of several factors, including the advocacy efforts of the profession itself. But the greatest impetus was generated as part of another progressive movement. This was the steady and increasingly rapid evolution of agriculture and of the farmers who practiced it. Both were becoming more sophisticated, a point emphasized by *The Ohio Farmer* in an editorial of January 6, 1883:

> In looking at the farmer today . . . a careful and honest comparison will show that he has in everything . . . made greater progress than men in almost any other calling in life . . . The farmer himself, as a man, has greatly improved. He reads and thinks more and no longer sneers at 'book' farming. A larger proportion of farmers belong to and sustain well a good organization, a grange or farmers' club. The farmers' institutes are not only well-attended, but many farmers are found among the lecturers at them. Agricultural colleges are now established in most, if not all of the states . . . Experimental stations are being established by both the state and by private individuals. . . . There has never been a time or a country where the calling of the farmer was more honored and respected than this.

Rural America was changing and veterinary medicine had the opportunity to benefit from it. It was this fact, perhaps as much as anything else, that led a small group of Ohio veterinarians to converge on Columbus July 24, 1883, to form the Ohio Veterinary Medical Association.

A later Ohio text published in 1879 by a professional veterinarian. The inclusion of a chapter on dog diseases is interesting since, in this period, small animal care was largely ignored. (Ohio Historical Society)

Homœopathic Veterinary Hand-Book,

For the Farmer, Stockman and Horse Owner.

Giving in plain, practical terms, description, symptoms and remedies for all diseases of the Horse, Ox, Sheep, Swine and Dog.

By J. W. Johnson, V. S.

Veterinary p— —four years' experience; — —epartment of Ohio Farm— —d Practical Farmer, P—

PUBLISH— —ER CO.,

DISEASES OF THE DOG.

DISTEMPER.

A contagious disease of which all dogs appear to carry the seeds in their system, accompanied with fever and derangement of most of the internal organs, and frequently ending in cholera, paralysis, inflammation of the lungs, etc. It is most common in pups during the concluding period of dentition, and in the spring and autumn, particularly the latter, but at no age or at no season is a dog exempt from its attack. The younger the dog, the better is the chance of recovery. Superior breeds suffer most.

Causes.—Contact with dogs having the disease, too much meat while young, cold. As the disease is latent in the system, a great variety of circumstances may cause it to develop itself. Dogs that are confined are more susceptible than those that are free to roam; those that are fed upon flesh suffer more than those that never taste it.

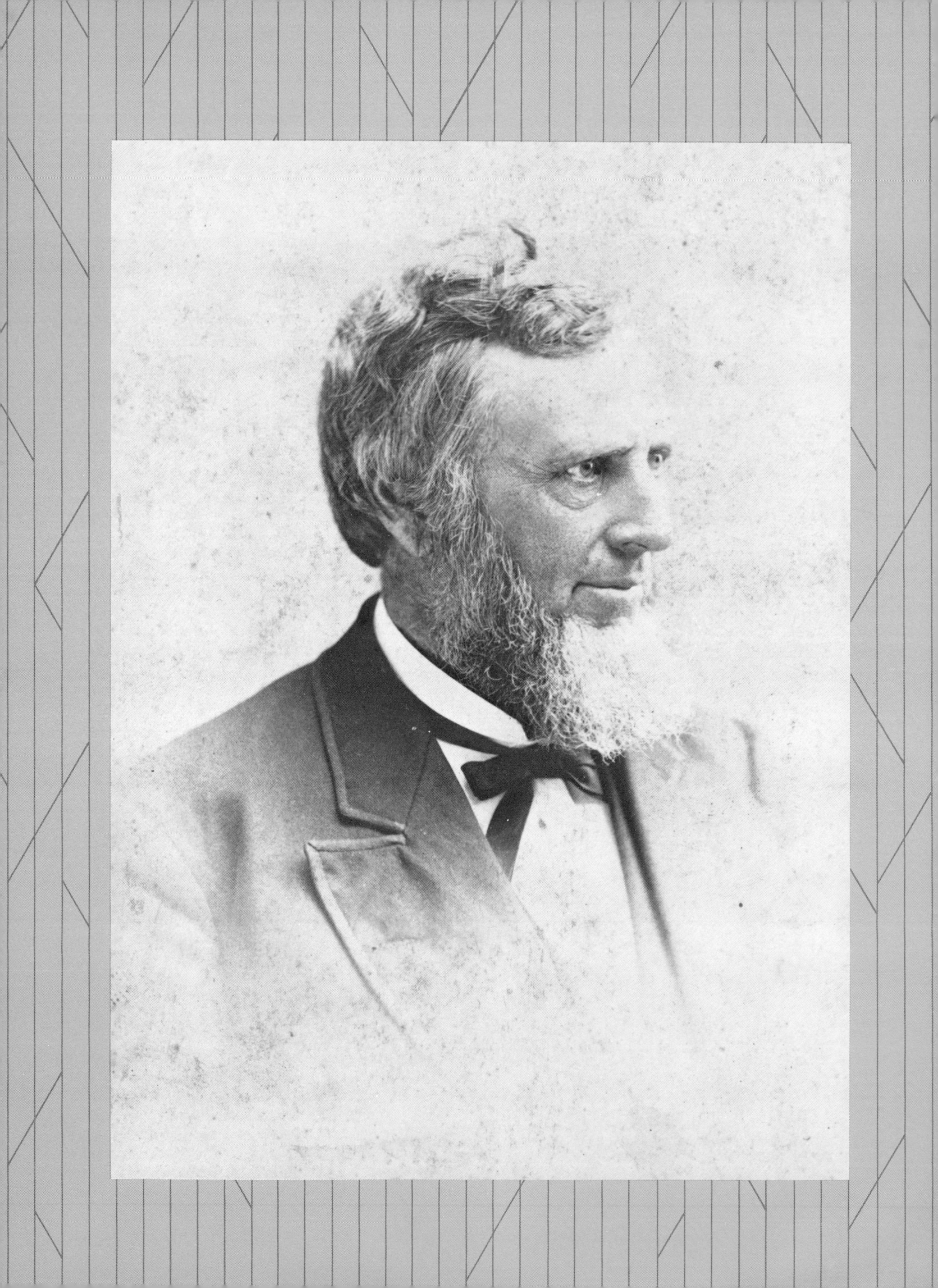

CHAPTER II

THE BIRTH OF THE OVMA

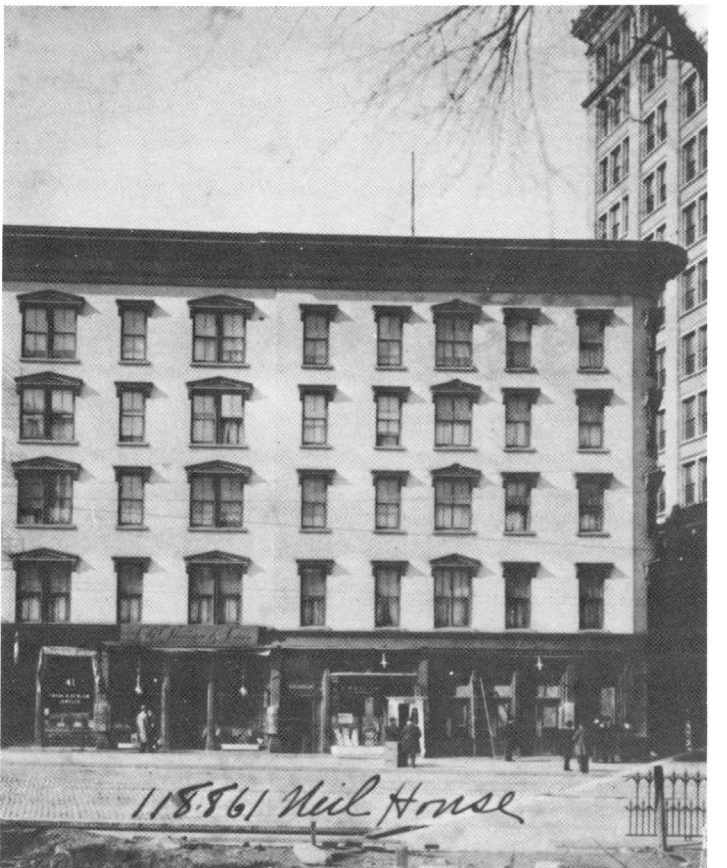

The Neil House as it appeared in the 1880s. Here, on July 24, 1883, a group of Ohio veterinarians met and "effected a permanent organization." (Ohio Historical Society)

Dr. Norton S. Townshend, M.D. A Renaissance man of Ohio agriculture, he championed scientific veterinary medicine and presided at the founding of the OVMA. (Photo Archives, Ohio State University)

Details of the founding of the Ohio Veterinary Medical Association are relatively sparse. They would be even sparser but for the foresight of Dr. F.A. Lambert, who served as secretary of the Association from 1915 to 1918. In 1916, concerned by the inadequacy of early records, he asked two veteran members to report at that year's annual meeting on the birth of the Association. One was Dr. John Newton of Toledo, a member of the organizing committee and a charter member; the other, Dr. Walter Shaw of Dayton, who joined the Association in 1885. The reports of these men, drawn from memory and fragmentary records, comprise the history of the founding of the OVMA and its earliest activities.

Dr. Newton, in his report, alluded to earlier discussions regarding formation of a veterinary association, and then described the first meeting:

> From time to time a few of us talked of organizing a state society, but all ended in talk, until the Spring of 1883, when a promoter, Mr. Daniels of Chicago, appeared on the scene, and through his personal solicitation and correspondence with the veterinarians of the state, a number of us assembled at the Neil House, Columbus, on Tuesday, July 24, 1883, at 2:30 p.m., for the purpose of organizing a State Veterinary Association. The following gentlemen were present to wit: T.B. Cotton, Mt. Vernon; A. Moor, Mansfield; J.C. Butler, Piqua; T.J. Marlin, (never qualified); W.E. Wight, Delaware; W.A. Labron, Xenia; V.A. Berry, Lima; T.B. Hillock, Columbus; J.S. Waddel, Columbus; J. Rose, Columbus; W.G. Jones, Delphi, Ohio; J. Bowersmith, Marysville. The meeting was called to order by Mr. Daniels of Chicago, who in a few well-chosen remarks, set forth the object of the meeting. Professor Townshend of OSU was elected Chairman, and T.B. Cotton, Secretary. On motion, the following gentlemen were appointed as committee on business: Cotton, Marlin, Butler, Moor, Waddel, Labron, Wight.

The meeting's first and most important order of business was to develop a constitution and by-laws. Quoting again from Dr. Newton's report:

> A recess was taken, committee retired for the consultation at 4:30 p.m. Committee reported a recommendation that constitution and by-laws of the Illinois State Veterinary Medical Association be adopted by this Association, with the exception of Article III, Section 1, 'Non-graduates, practicing five years can duly become a member by passing the Board of Censors.' On motion the report was received. Report of committee was

then discussed. On motion the amended Constitution and By-Laws of Illinois State Veterinary Medical Association were adopted for the government of this Association.

This would indicate that the new Assocation intended from the very beginning to admit to membership only graduate veterinarians. But a 1904 report contradicts this view; in a brief historical summary that year, Secretary William H. Gribble said that graduates and non-graduates alike were eligible for membership at the time of the Association's founding and that a change in the by-laws restricting future membership to graduates was not made until 1889. Since records are so fragmentary, it is impossible to resolve the conflict; suffice to say that early on the OVMA did begin restricting membership to graduates of veterinary schools.

The next order of business at the first meeting was the election of officers, the names of whom are listed in the *Dispatch* story. Mr. Daniels and Professor Townshend were then elected honorary members of the Association, after which the names of eight veterinarians were presented and all of them elected to membership. With that, the first meeting of the OVMA drew to a close.

> A vote of thanks was tendered Professor Townshend and Mr. Daniels of Chicago for their valuable services rendered in the organizing of this Association. Adjourned to meet again at Union Hall, Ohio State Fair Grounds, on the 5th day of September, 1883, at 2 p.m. sharp.

The two men thanked and accorded honorary membership in the fledgling OVMA deserve attention; both played significant roles in the Association's founding.

"Mr. Daniels of Chicago" was T.D. Daniels, a promoter with a strong interest in veterinary medicine. At the time of his trip to Columbus, he was promoting the formation of veterinary associations throughout the middle and western states, and the publication of a veterinary journal which he intended to start in Chicago. The two efforts were obviously linked and Daniels actively solicited support for his proposed journal at the first meeting of the OVMA. As Dr. Newton recalled in his 1916 report:

> ... it was a flowery story that good man told us as to the good it would do the profession and would pay great dividends to its stockholders. Shares of $500.00 each were issued ... Several of our Charter members purchased shares and have the certificates among our archives of the past. The *Journal* did not live long and years ago Mr. Daniels died—peace to his ashes and rest to his soul. I believe his motives were all right, and had he lived to be present at this meeting he would have felt he had his reward—if not in dollars in the great work accomplished by the O.S.V.M.A. . . .

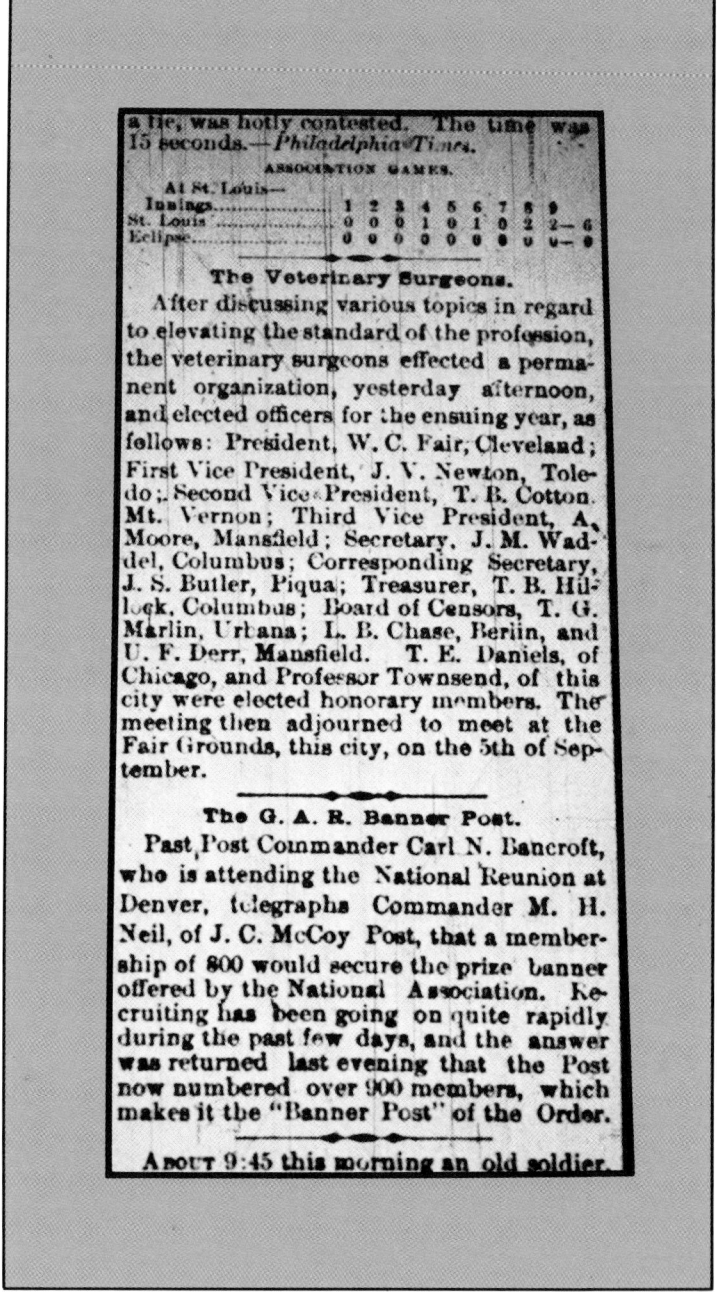

The press takes note. The first story in the Columbus Dispatch, *July 25, 1883. (Ohio Historical Society)*

There is no evidence that Daniels was anything but sincere in his promotion of veterinary associations and his journal. While the latter did not survive, he did help achieve something of much greater permanence and importance in Ohio; it was his "personal solicitation and correspondence with the veterinarians of the state" that brought the founders of the OVMA to Columbus.

If Daniels was the prime generator of activity in 1883, the second honorary member of the OVMA was the man whose long-term efforts had created a

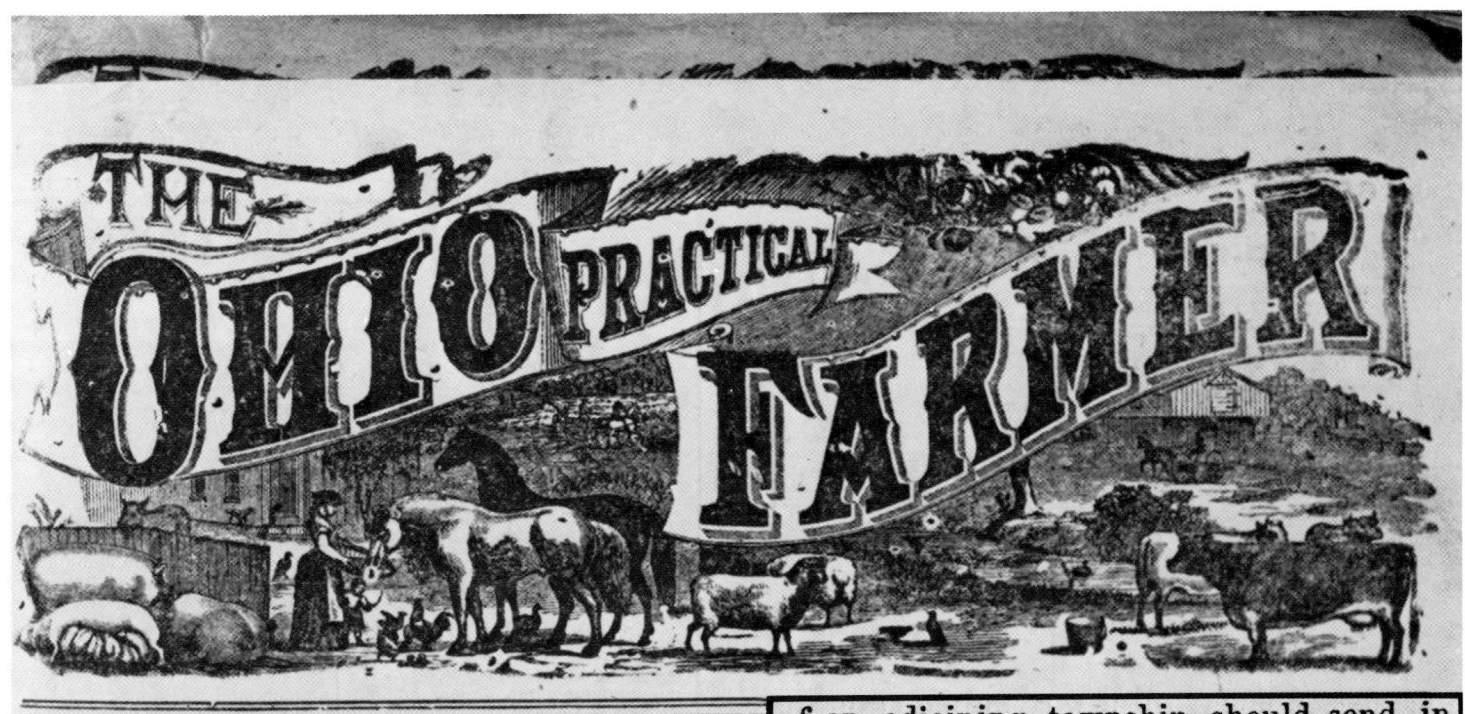

climate in which action could take place. "Professor Townshend of this city," as he was identified by *The Columbus Dispatch*, was Norton Strange Townshend, M.D., a practical visionary who was truly a Renaissance man of Ohio agriculture.

Born in England in 1815, Townshend migrated to the United States with his parents in 1830 and settled on a farm at Avon in Ohio's Lorain County. He became a practitioner of human medicine and also developed an ardent interest in agriculture, particularly animal husbandry. In time, this interest would dominate his activities; Townshend became a pioneer in scientific agriculture, one of the founders of The Ohio State University, and its first professor of agriculture. He also established himself as one of the strongest advocates of scientific veterinary medicine, believing that trained veterinary practitioners were essential for the maintenance of a healthy livestock industry.

Dr. Townshend's contributions to the development of veterinary science will be covered in more detail in the section on the OSU College of Veterinary Medicine. For now, it is enough to say that those contributions resulted in the steady advance of the veterinary profession and paved the way for the founding of the state association. No more appropriate person could have been chosen to chair the organizing meeting.

As Dr. Newton reports, the newly formed OVMA scheduled a second session for September, 1883;

The OVMA's second meeting as reported in The Ohio Farmer, *September 15, 1883. The Association and its activities were not yet front page news. (Ohio Historical Society)*

Columbus, Ohio, in the early 1880s. (Ohio Historical Society)

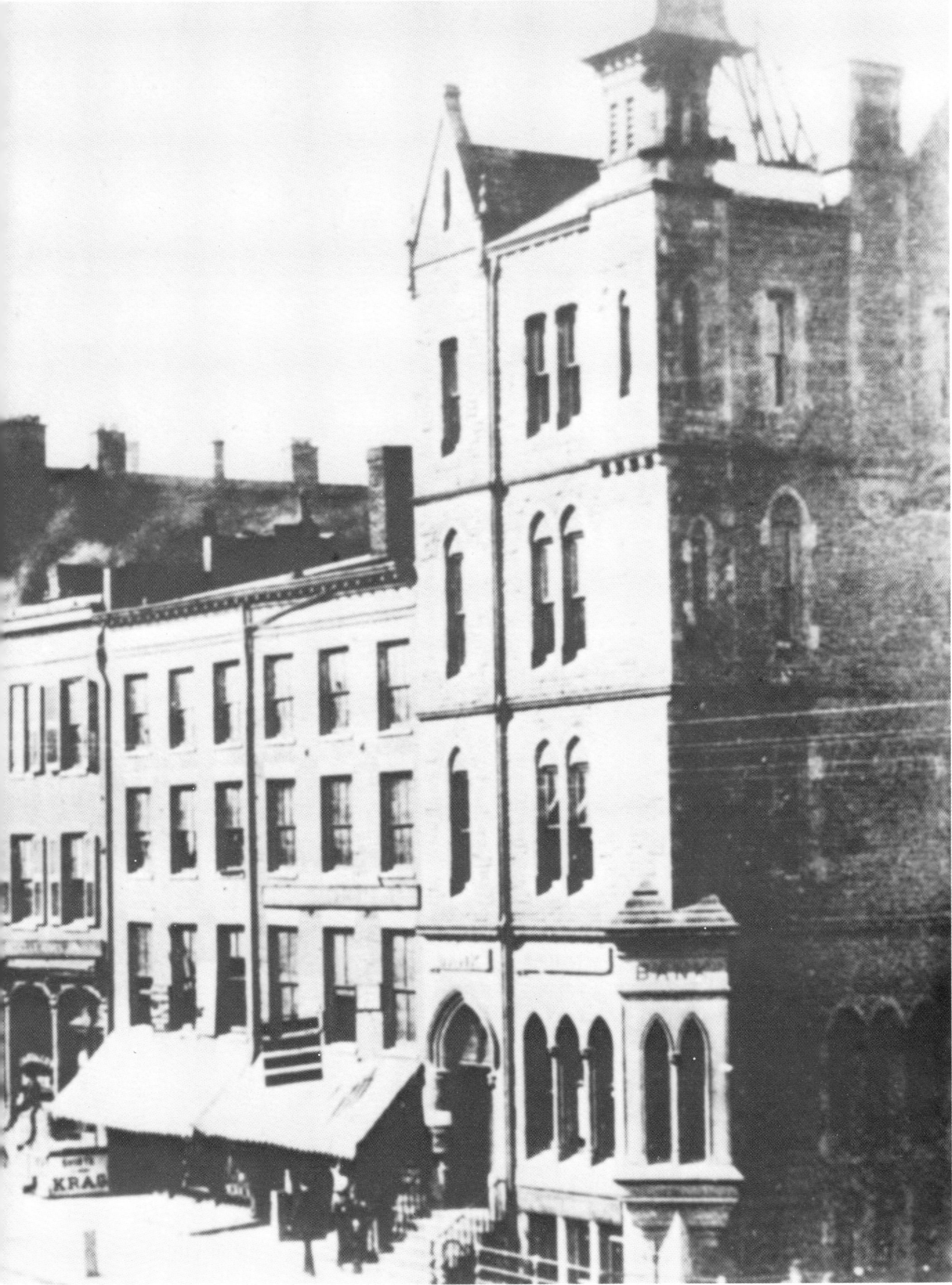

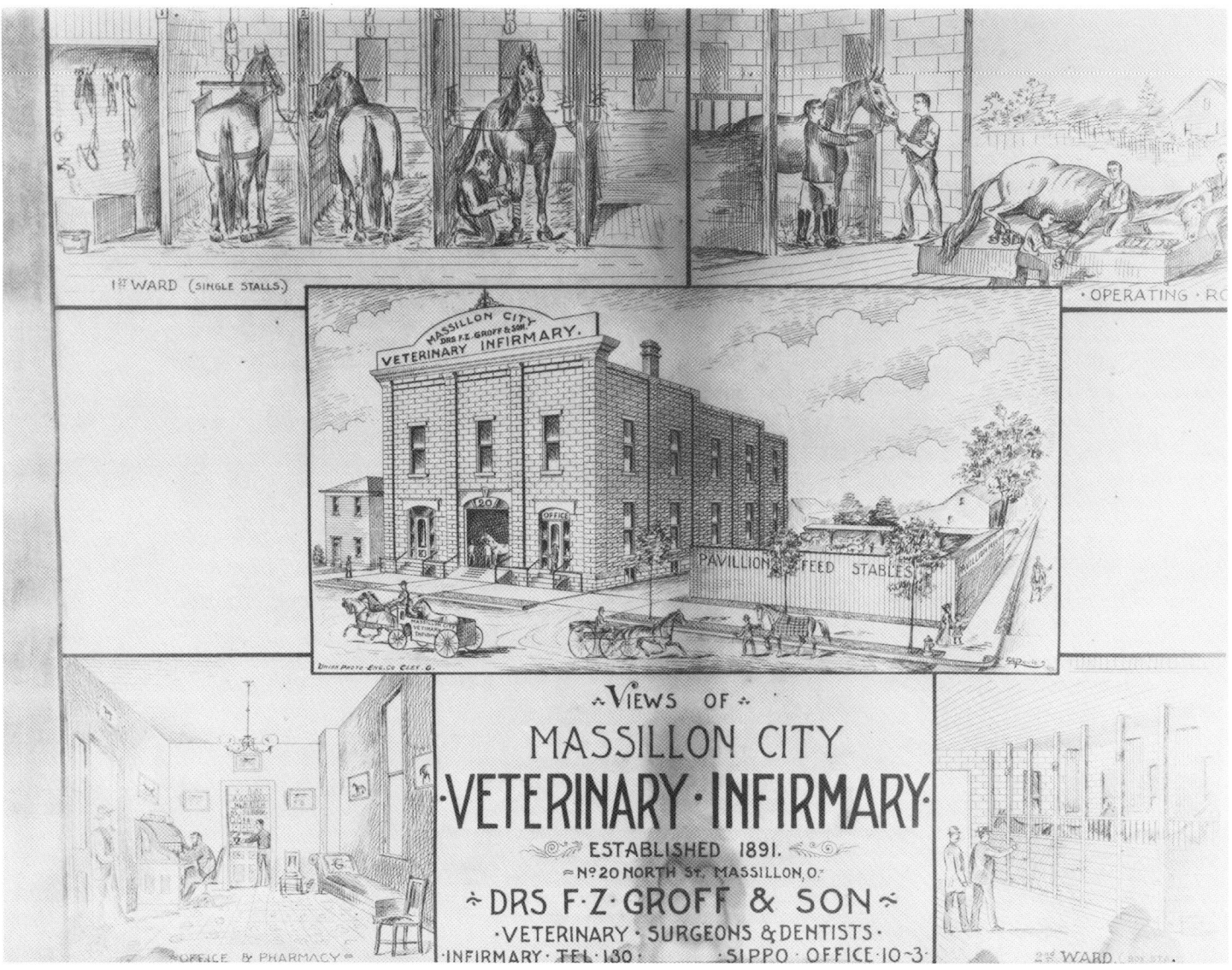

The growth of professional veterinary medicine was sometimes frustratingly slow. But in 1891 Massillon could boast the services of a complete Veterinary Infirmary. The emphasis was clearly on horses. (Picture: Dr. Charles Beutel)

clearly the founders were interested in sustaining momentum. This one drew the attention of *The Ohio Farmer,* which carried a brief story in its September 15 issue:

> A meeting of the Ohio State Veterinary Association was held on the (State Fair) grounds on Wednesday, Dr. Fair of Cleveland presiding. There were fifteen members present. The meeting was an interesting one, however, and a number of important subjects were discussed. It was decided to admit none to the association but regular graduates of veterinary or other medical schools.

The *Farmer* story further muddies the admissions picture. Also, Dr. Newton, in his 1916 report on the same meeting, writes:

The applications of some *graduates* to become members were referred to the Board of Censors and laid over to the next meeting. Moved and seconded that Dr. Howe be appointed in Mr. Marlin's place on the Board of Censors, as Mr. Marlin, being a non-graduate, could not act.

The Newton report of 1916 also provides additional details on the OVMA's second session. He notes that "bills of printing books and cards were ordered paid.... A lively discussion followed in regard to Veterinary Dentistry by Dr. Cotton, who promised for the next meeting a paper on the above subject. Dr. Hawkins of Detroit was then called upon and made a few remarks in regards to Veterinary Associations . . . (and) Professor Townshend was then called upon, but declined to speak because of the lateness of the hour. After spending a pleasant afternoon, the meeting then closed to meet again in Cleveland, second Tuesday in January, 1884."

The Ohio Farmer did *not* cover the Association's next meeting which was held on January 8. But it did carry a story on January 19, couched in somewhat waspish tones:

> We learn from the daily papers that the Ohio State Veterinary Association held a meeting in this city January 8, with an attendance of about 35 members. This paper never received a notice of the meeting or we would have had a representative present to record any information of value brought out. We notice that Dr. Fair, the president, asserted that... children who drank the milk of cattle (with tuberculosis) were likely to contract lung disease. Dr. Cotton said that wolf teeth (in horses) caused disease of the eyes, often terminating in blindness, but this was denied by others present. The only other questions discussed according to the *Leader's* report, was 'rumpture of the diaphragm', something not 'down in the books' and 'lockjaw', a disease that veterinary surgeons never suffer from. The next meeting will be held at Toledo during the June races.

Hell hath no fury like a journalist ignored.

Again, we are indebted to Dr. Newton for a more complete report on the January 8 session, which was designated the Second Annual Meeting. In addition to commenting on the presentations of Dr. Fair and Dr. Cotton, he notes that:

> Dr. Bowler of Cincinnati... made a few remarks in regard to progress of Veterinary Surgery, the doctor being veterinary surgeon to the Zoological Gardens of Cincinnati, making wild animals a special study. He gave a short history of the elephant, also castration of and the danger of peritonitis in same.... Dr. Hillock related a very interesting case of Diaphragmatic Hernia which showed symptoms of acute indigestion.... President Fair reported a case of Tetanus which ended in death. Dr. Newton then introduced the subject, parturient apoplexy, after which a lively discussion followed. Dr. Derr volunteered a paper on apoplexy at our next meeting. Dr. Whitehead promised one on tuberculosis.

Dr. Newton concluded his 1916 report by observing that "This is what our records show as to the founding and early meetings of our Association." Admittedly, those records are fragmentary and much of the early history is lost. But a review of Dr. Newton's brief summary makes it clear that, from the very beginning, there was an impressive emphasis on continuing education and a sharing of knowledge by the members of the OVMA. Their profession was serious business and so was their new Association.

There was also strong emphasis on professional ethics. Dr. Walter Shaw of Dayton, the second veteran to present a historical report at the 1916 Annual meeting, focused on this early in his presentation, telling members:

> I first attended a meeting of this Association December 26, 1885. There were twelve members present and charges were preferred against two to expel them for non-professional conduct. One was expelled, the other laid over until the following meeting in June... when he was expelled. After this charges were laid against a prominent member for taking a special course in veterinary dentistry and advertising it, but owing to the doctor's political experience, his ability as a vote getter, and his great personality, he was able to escape with a suspended sentence.... A year later the most prominent veterinarian in the state at that time was expelled because he recommend Gombold's Caustic Balsam to cure colic in a calf. This procedure continued for some time and though it may seem radical, no doubt had a good effect.

Thin as its ranks were in those early years, the OVMA did not hesitate to purge from them unethical practitioners. At the same time, obviously, it was equally interested in attracting qualified, ethical veterinarians. But, like all new groups, it faced problems, a major one being the peripatetic character of its meetings. Again, quoting Dr. Shaw:

> From the beginning the Association traveled around for several years from one town or city to another with the view to getting new members, which was not always successful. If a new member was secured in the northern portion of the state he would not attend the next meeting in the southwestern portion or some equally remote corner. Therefore he would soon be dropped for non-payment of dues or some other cause, so the growth of the Association was slow.

In one five year period, 1886-1890, Association meetings were held in ten different cities and, while there may have been some merit to moving about, the practice also was an obstacle to permanence and cohesion. The issue was finally resolved in 1890, although not everyone was happy with the solution. As Dr. Shaw reported:

> From January, 1890, the annual meetings were held in Columbus in January. The summer meetings convened in different places as a sort of sweep net to catch new members. While the an-

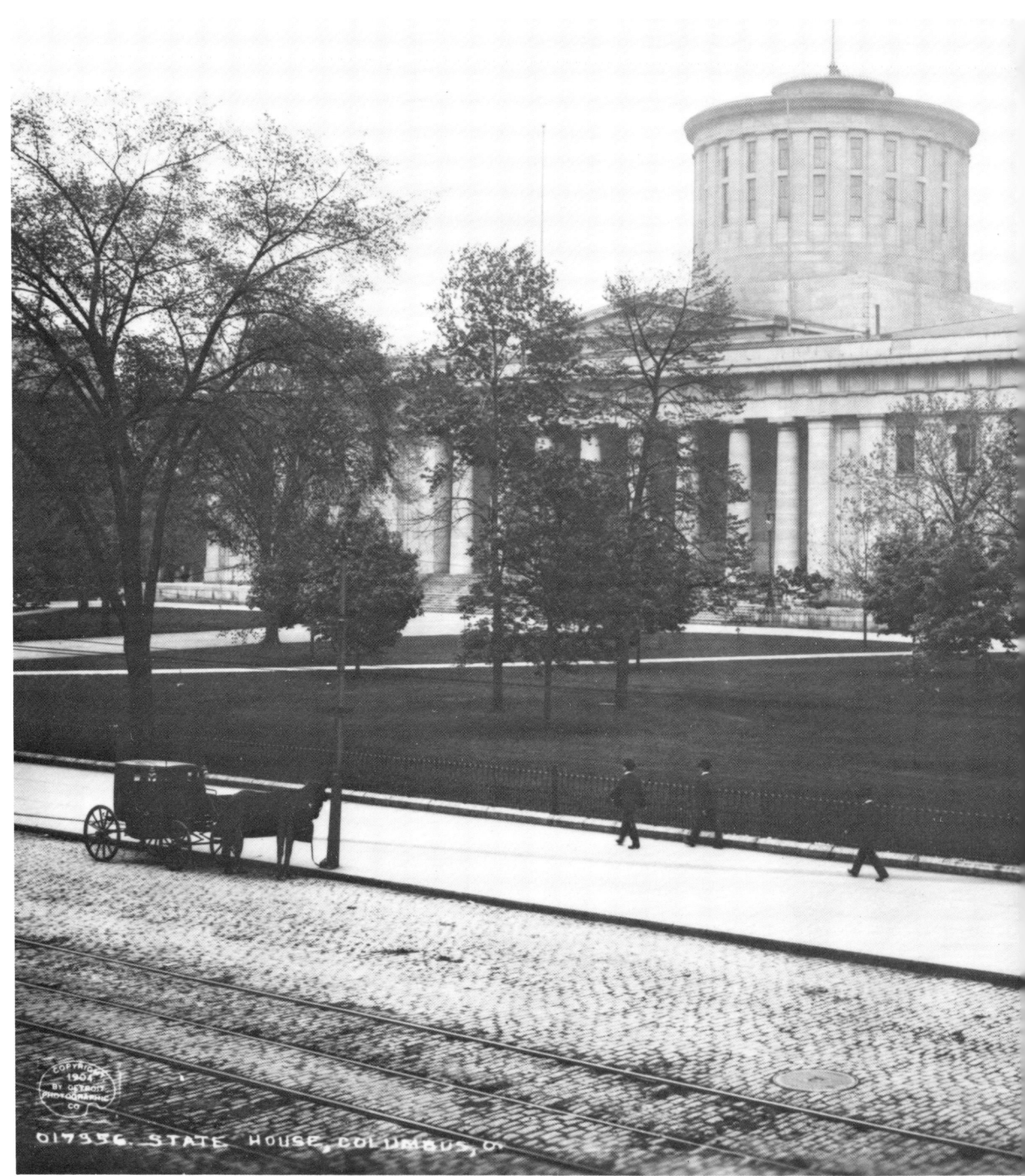

Early in the campaign against quackery, the OVMA sought legislation licensing veterinary practice. But several years passed before a Practice Act finally cleared the State Legislature. (Ohio Historical Society)

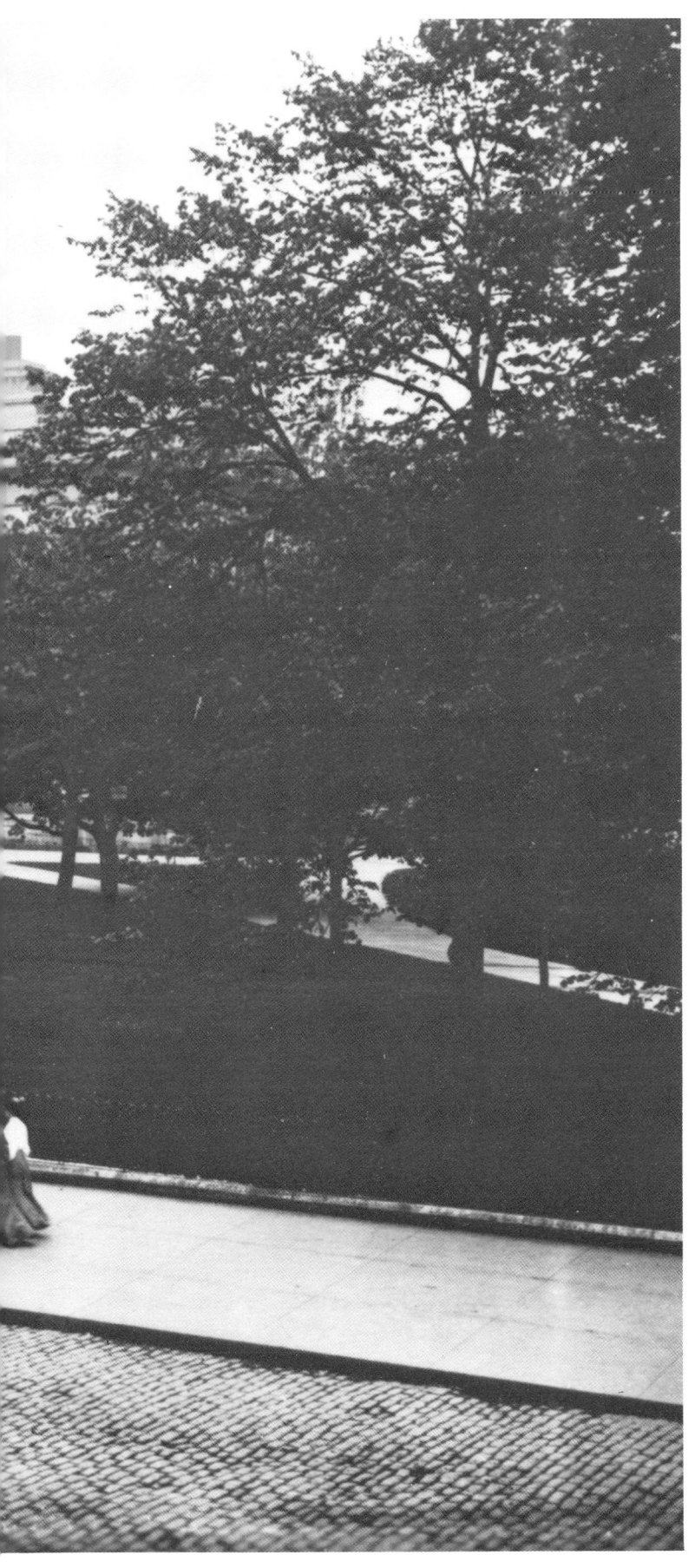

nual meetings were held in Columbus, it was done with some difficulty, some inexperienced members wishing to convert it again to a caravan. In 1904, the constitution was changed and located the annual meeting permanently in Columbus. . . . After the Association was permanently located, its membership began a permanent growth. . . .

The problem of meeting location was solved relatively early in the Association's history. But another obstacle to membership would take much longer to surmount. This involved the status of untrained practitioners—the "quacks" who still outnumbered graduate veterinarians ten to one. Dr. Shaw observed that many trained practitioners were waiting to see what the new Association was going to do about them:

> When a veterinarian was asked to join the Association he would often say, 'The Association has done nothing. When it has a law passed to stop the quacks from practicing, I will join.'

This attitude, prevailing among many badly-needed potential members, obviously had an impact on the OVMA, as did the validity of the concern. So it is no surprise that one of the Association's earliest actions was to mount a campaign against quackery and unlicensed practice.

It was a campaign that would go on for years.

The OVMA's first major assault on quackery took it into the chambers of the Ohio Legislature. To Association leaders, it was apparent that the quickest way to eliminate untrained and self-appointed practitioners would be to pass legislation licensing the practice of veterinary medicine. Many of the "doctors of animals" would be unable to pass the required examination and they would be effectively outlawed and out-of-business.

But this approach, while the quickest, was far from easy. Untrained "medicine men" heavily outnumbered professional veterinarians and they had political clout. Moreover, there was disagreement among Association members about the campaign. The result was that early efforts to pass legislation ended in failure, as Dr. Shaw reported in 1916:

> At the annual meeting January 11, 1887, it was deemed advisable to appoint a committee . . . to draft a bill to regulate the practice of veterinary medicine and surgery in Ohio. . . . A very good bill was drafted, which required all persons who had not been in practice in the state for three years preceding its passage, who wished to practice in the state to pass an examination as to his qualifications. A number of graduated veteri-

narians in the state who had passed one examination and objected to passing another, opposed this clause and the bill was lost. Since the veterinarians in the state were unable to agree, future bills met the same fate, until Professor Detmers got one passed in 1894.

Professor Detmers was H.J. Detmers, the first Professor of Veterinary Medicine at Ohio State University and in 1894, Chief of the OSU Veterinary School. He is one of the most significant figures in Ohio veterinary history and there will be more on his career in the section on education.

The bill shaped by Detmers and maneuvered through the Ohio Legislature (H.B. 335) mandated that "all persons who now, or shall hereafter, practice veterinary medicine and surgery in the state of Ohio, and have not been engaged in such practice for at least three years prior to the passage of this act, in the state of Ohio, shall be examined as to their qualifications by a state board of veterinary examiners, to be appointed as hereinafter provided.... A certificate shall be issued only when the board is satisfied that the candidate examined is well qualified and entitled to a certificate."

It was a partial victory. To a degree, veterinary medicine was now regulated in Ohio. And the regulation was achieved three years before passage of a similar law governing the practice of Human Medicine, a fact that reportedly led one newspaper to observe that "In Ohio not every man can treat a Jackass, but any Jackass can treat a man."

In light of this it is interesting to note that a doctor of human medicine, Van S. Deaton, played a key role in the passage of the first veterinary practice act. A state representative from Miami County, Dr. Deaton actually wrote the bill and fought for it in the legislature. A commendatory reference in the OVMA's 1915-16 Yearbook says:

> He has often been rightly referred to as the legislative Father of the Veterinary Profession in Ohio. He was the author in 1894 of the first veterinary practice act in the state, and in 1915 was the guardian of our interests when the rewritten law was passed. No citizen of Ohio has proven himself a better friend of the veterinary profession than has Dr. Deaton.

But while the 1894 law was a significant achievement, it was not perfect. The language of the bill "grandfathered in" both graduates and nongraduates who had been practicing veterinary medicine for at least three years prior to its passage, which meant that these people were entitled to certificates without an examination. So while the bill gave new legal status to professionally-trained veterinarians, it

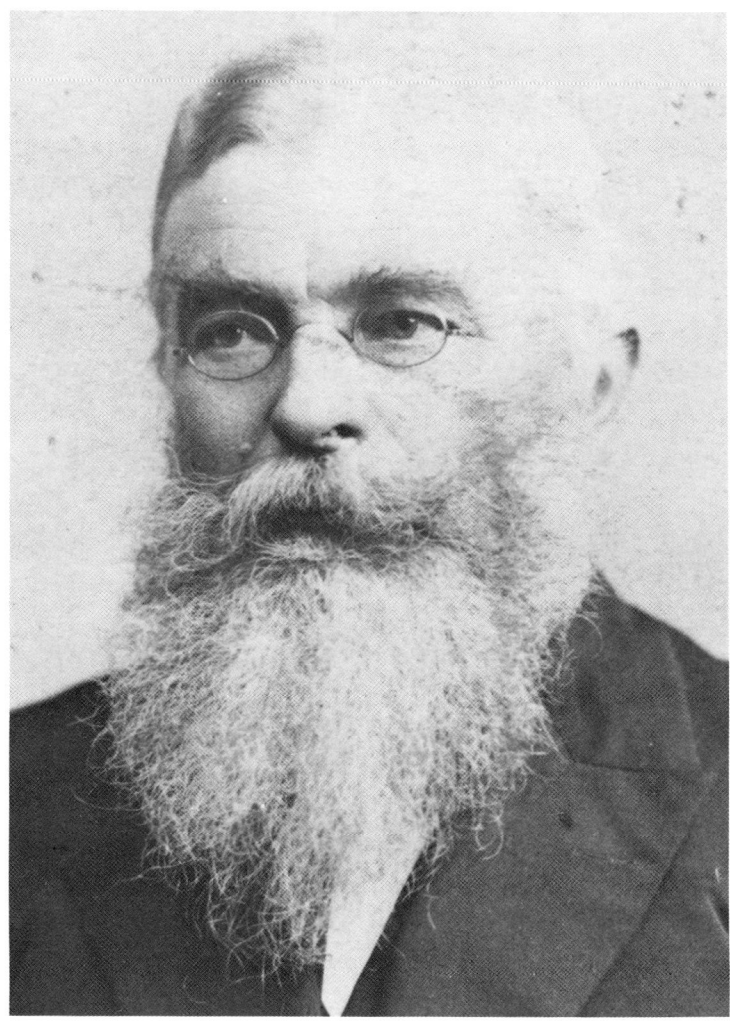

Dr. H. J. Detmers, the first Professor of Veterinary Medicine at Ohio State University and the architect of Ohio's first Veterinary Practice Act. (Photo Archives, Ohio State University)

allowed many untrained practitioners to continue in business, also with legal status.

And continue they did, to the increasing dissatisfaction of the OVMA. Nearly twenty years after passage of the Practice Act, the Association was as deeply involved as ever in its antiquackery campaign. The first Yearbook, reporting on the Annual Meeting for 1911-12, included a devastating broadside aimed at untrained and incompetent practitioners:

> The Ohio State Veterinary Medical Association is Striving to Eradicate Veterinary Quackery, because Veterinary Quackery Menaces the Public Health, Greatly Increases Live Stock Losses, and Is Responsible for Much Avoidable Suffering in Animals.

> The inability and failure of the competent veterinarian to recognize in his patients such diseases of animals as are transmissible to man causes needless exposure of all persons coming in contact with such animals and not infrequently re-

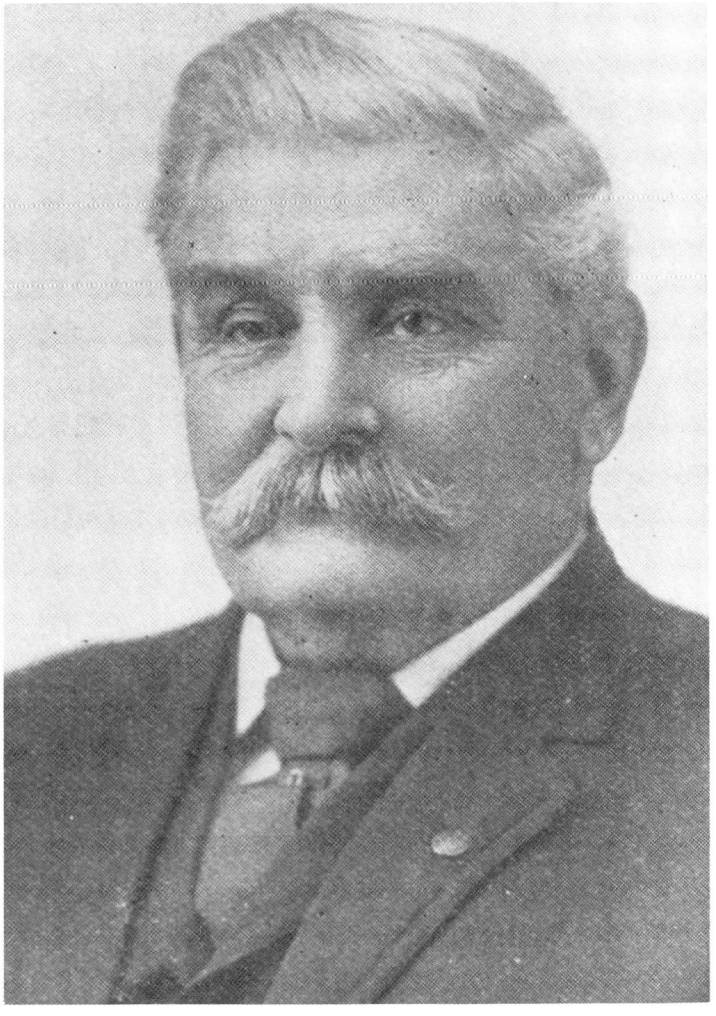

Dr. Van S. Deaton, M.D., and State Representative. The "Legislative Father of the Veterinary Profession in Ohio." (OVMA files)

sults in human infection with serious or fatal results.... Many animals, suffering with curable diseases or injuries, are lost through the inability of the incompetent veterinarian.... It is safe to say that incompetent veterinarians are responsible for the annual loss of millions of dollars invested in Ohio live-stock.... Through lack of skill incompetent veterinary practitioners cause and prolong animal suffering.... When the people of Ohio who are interested in the State's health and live stock interests and who feel for the suffering animal realize the importance and value of efficient veterinary service and the dangers of veterinary quackery, they will encourage veterinary education and condemn veterinary quackery and insist upon the strict enforcement of the State law regulating the practice of veterinary medicine and surgery.

In this blistering indictment, the Association denied any ulterior motive, noting that quacks did not cut into the practice of qualified veterinarians:

... on the contrary they, by their bungling attempts at surgery and by their mistakes in diagnosis and in the improper use of drugs, actually make and increase the practice and business of the qualified veterinarian. The Association therefore cannot be accused of selfish motives in its warfare on quackery.

The records indicate that the campaign against quackery was particularly intense in this period; there are numerous and lengthy references to the issue in Association Yearbooks. Addressing the 1912-13 Annual Meeting, Association President Dr. L.P. Cook reported on an effort to water down the Practice Act and the Association's response:

Since our last annual meeting your officers were called upon to resist a determined effort on the part of politicians to amend the law regulating the practice of veterinary medicine in this state. The two bills seeking to amend the law which were pending at the time of our last meeting were, through the efforts of your officers and the State Board of Veterinary Examiners and a few members, killed in committee. The passage of either of these bills would have been disastrous to your profession.

It was a reminder to members that what one legislative session had wrought, another session could dismantle. Protection of the Practice Act would remain high on the OVMA's action agenda for years to come.

In the same address, President Cook also discussed another area of Association involvement, equally direct:

Every known illegal practitioner was warned of the intention of the Association to enforce the Law. This warning was more effective than expected. Though not a single prosecution was made, several hundred illegal practitioners promptly discontinued practice.... To my mind, this warfare on quackery should go on unrelentingly.

The 1912–13 Annual Meeting also took action in response to a related problem. This involved fake veterinary correspondence schools in Ohio which were selling bogus diplomas and swelling the ranks of quackery. To curb the practice, the Association passed a resolution directing the President to advertise through newspapers and otherwise "the fact that correspondence school diplomas do not give the holder any right to practice veterinary medicine, surgery or dentistry and that no correspondence school graduate has ever passed an examination before the State Board of Veterinary Examiners of Ohio." The sum of $100 was appropriated for the advertisements.

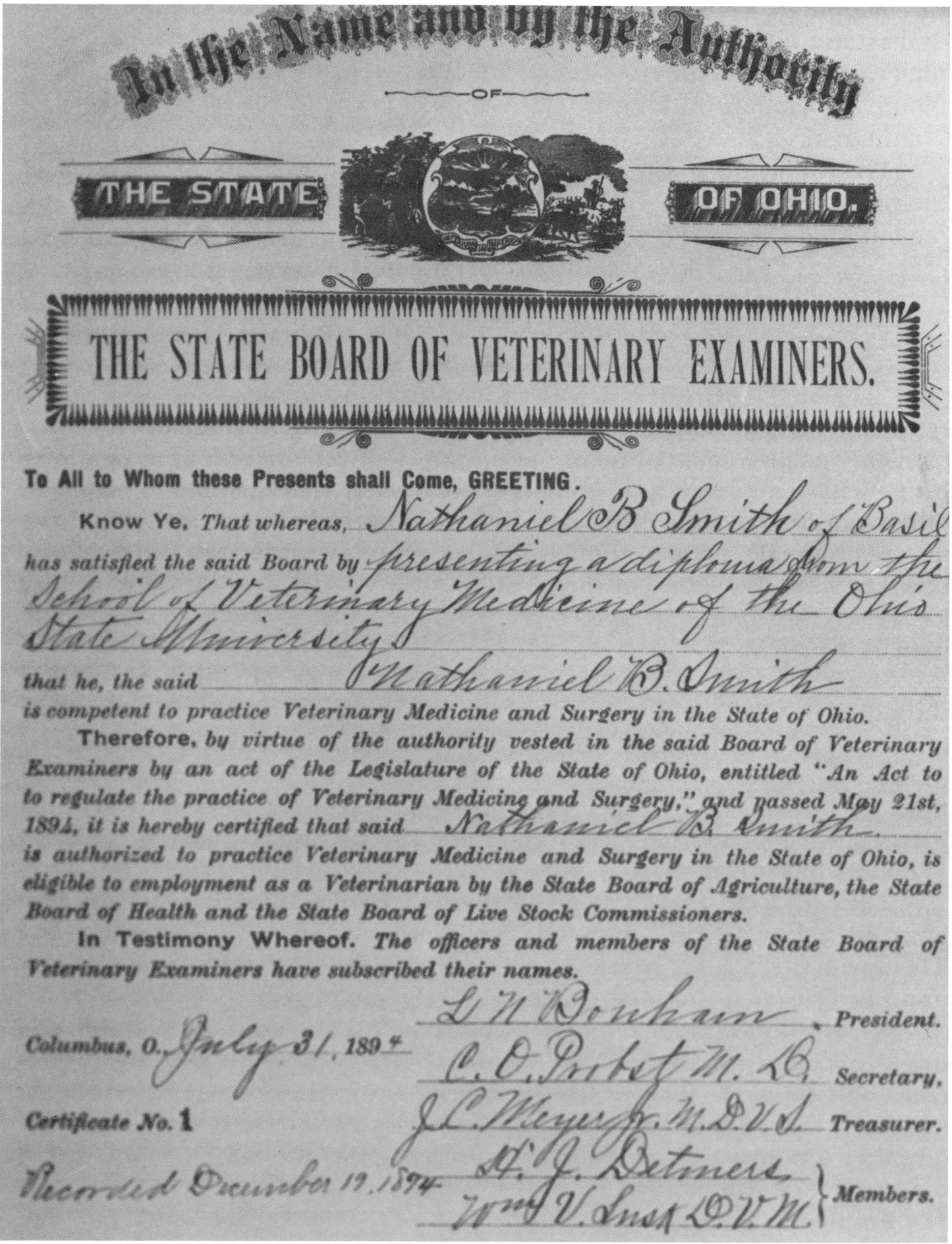

In succeeding years the problem of quackery became more manageable. Attrition thinned the ranks of non-graduates "grandfathered" into legal practice and there were successful efforts to strengthen Practice legislation, all strongly supported by the OVMA.

The Ohio Legislature passed a new Practice Act in 1925, H.B. 429. It required that applicants for state examination be graduates of veterinary colleges recognized by the Board of Veterinary Examiners, but did not apply to "those persons already duly licensed under the laws of the state." This Act was amended in 1936; the criteria for an applicant was rewritten to read that they "shall be a graduate of a veterinary college having standards and requirements equal to the standards and requirements of the Veterinary College of Ohio State University." In 1958, this was changed again; applicants for examination were required to have "obtained an education from a veterinary college approved by the Board (of Veterinary Examiners)."

The evolution of the Practice Act steadily elevated the quality of professional veterinary medicine in Ohio. But it did not totally eliminate quackery; after all, it is one thing to pass a law, quite another to enforce it. While quackery was waning, unlicensed practitioners remained in business and sometimes it was hard to get at them. A report at the Association's 1929 Annual Meeting noted the continuing difficulty:

> There have been a few attempts made within the state to prosecute, but none successfully . . . (the problem being) "the difficulty of collecting evidence that will stand up in court."

At the same meeting, F.A. Zimmer, former State Veterinarian, cited problems in trying to prosecute through the State Board of Examiners, telling members that in many instances political pressure was brought to bear to protect illegal practitioners. Zimmer, who would later serve as OVMA president, proposed that the Association employ its own attorneys to obtain evidence and prosecute. In response, members appropriated $250 for this purpose.

The Association continued this direct involvement through the 1930s. In 1937, it set up a Practice Act Enforcement Committee, hiring its own investigator and selecting attorneys at various points in the state to prosecute cases. The investigator was Charles O. Roshon of Pataskala, retained at a salary of $25 a week, plus four cents a mile for the use of his car and traveling expenses. All indications are that Roshon did an effective job; the Enforcement Committee would later report that between October, 1937, and January, 1939, 26 people were prosecuted for illegal practice. And at the Annual Meeting in 1938, the Association authorized the Executive Committee "to set up a budget for the continuation of the program for the enforcement of the Practice Act which will include the employment of an investigator and attorneys as needed."

With this program, the OVMA was in effect assuming a quasi-governmental role, taking on a job that the under-funded Board of Veterinary Examiners could not handle. Later, for a brief period, the Association provided funds directly to the Board for Practice Act enforcement, but this cooperative effort was struck down by a legal opinion. Since then, the OVMA has concentrated its efforts on securing adequate public funding for the Veterinary Board.

Today, with quackery an insignificant problem and the word itself almost quaint, it may seem that the OVMA sometimes overreacted to the problem posed by illegal practitioners. But quackery was a very legitimate concern; Association leaders recognized from the very first that the progress of professional veterinary medicine would be impeded so long as self-appointed "healers" shared its domain. So the campaign against quackery, long and often arduous, was also very necessary and it ranks as a major achievement of the OVMA.

But not the only one. Equally important are the Association's contributions to quality veterinary education.

Ohio's first license to practice veterinary medicine, issued to Nathaniel B. Smith of Basil. (OVMA files)

As noted in the text, one of the milestones in the development of professional veterinary medicine in the United States was the founding in 1863 of the United States Veterinary Medical Association, now the American Veterinary Medical Association (AVMA). After organizing in 1883, the Ohio Veterinary Medical Association formed a close working relationship with the national group, benefiting from its advocacy of the profession and contributing to it the leadership services of many prominent OVMA members. Five Ohio veterinarians have served as president of the AVMA, beginning with Dr. David S. White, who was elected in 1920. Subsequent AVMA presidents from Ohio include Dr. Reuben Hilty, 1927–28; Dr. O. V. Brumley, 1937–38; Dr. R. E. Rebrassier, 1958–59; and Dr. Vernon Tharp, who headed the national association in 1978.

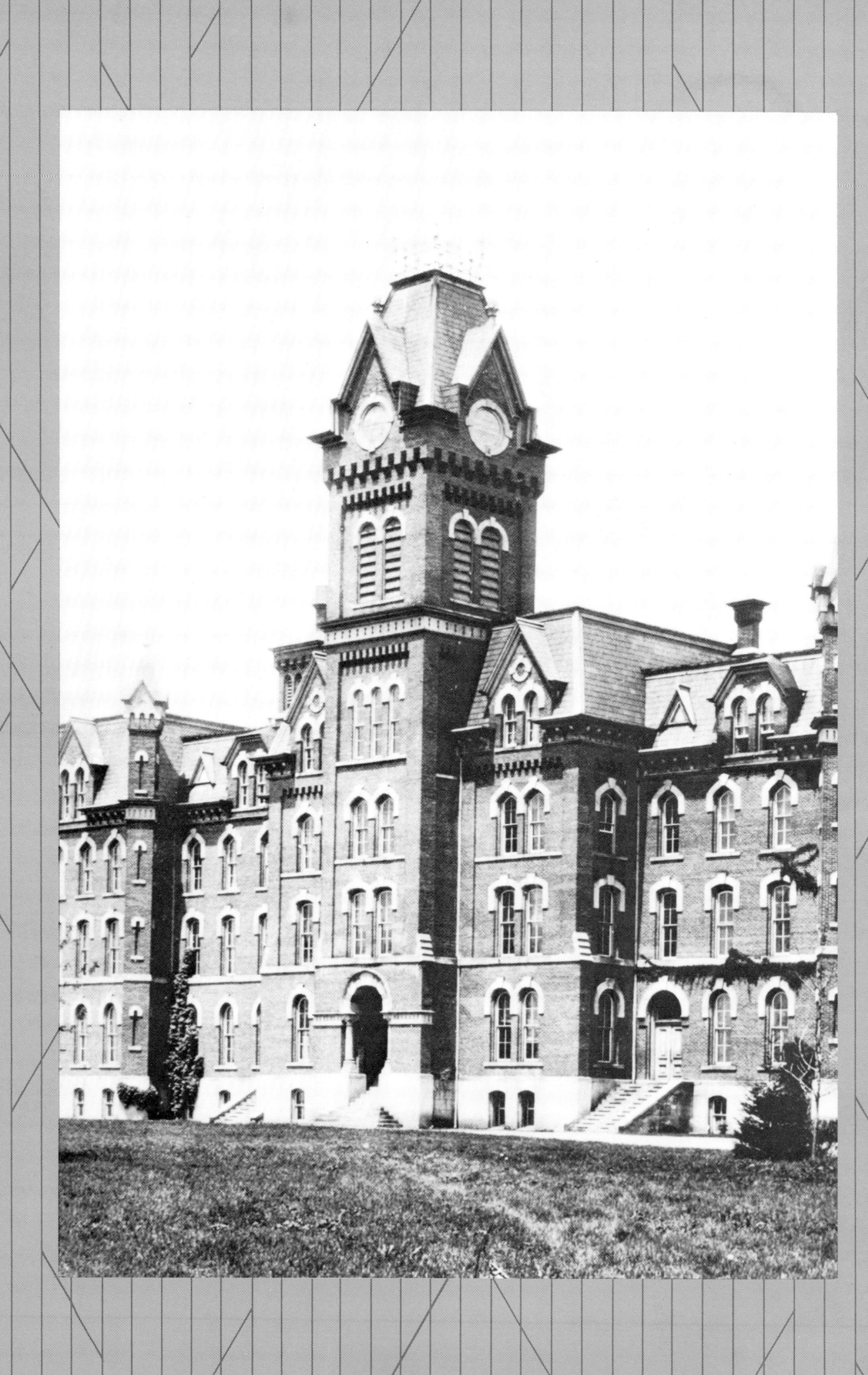

CHAPTER III

THE GROWTH OF EDUCATION

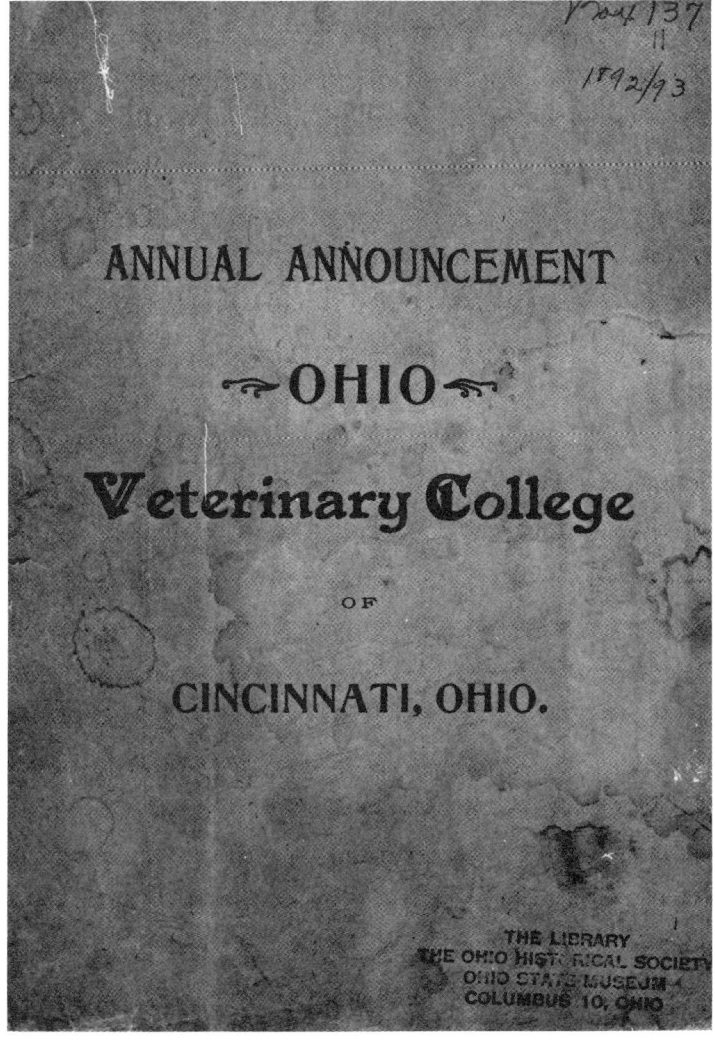

The 1892-93 Annual Announcement of the Ohio Veterinary College, the state's first important private veterinary school. It was in operation from 1891 to 1896. (Ohio Historical Society)

In the beginning there were the private schools. For several decades from the mid-1800s on, they were the good and bad custodians of veterinary education in the United States, springing up in the absence of state-supported schools and then, by their very presence, impeding the latter's development. This was particularly true in the late 1800s when the continued growth of private schools paralleled the growth of land grant colleges and their schools of agriculture. In "A Short History of Veterinary Medicine in America," B.W. Bierer writes:

> Private veterinary schools developing during the same period acted as deterrents to the development of the agricultural veterinary colleges... the private veterinary schools delayed the development of veterinary schools in some of the state agricultural schools for more than 50 years.

Bierer also noted that many of the private colleges were urban-oriented and responded primarily to the growing veterinary needs of America's larger cities.

> (These) private veterinary schools evolved to supply the wants and needs which largely stemmed from the ever-increasing demands for horse power, created by the rapidly-expanding industrial revolution in America. The private veterinary schools were established and flourished as horse power became more and more important.

The record of private veterinary education in Ohio includes an 1855 announcement by the Ohio Agricultural College of Cleveland of its second session "with instruction given in lectures... to include Comparative Anatomy and Physiology... (and) Veterinary Medicine." But it was not until the 1890s that Ohio had a noteworthy private school; in the state's history there would be only two, both located in Cincinnati. Both were also founded after the development of veterinary medical education at Ohio State University and thus were never serious deterrents to public education.

University Hall, better known as "Old Main" in 1887. Veterinary medicine was taught here, as were the other courses offered by what was originally The Ohio Agricultural and Mechanical College. It was the college's first and, for a time, only building. (Photo Archives, Ohio State University)

The first of these private schools was the Ohio Veterinary College of Cincinnati. Founded in 1891, it remained in operation until 1896, graduating in that period 67 men. The college offered a two-year course, with about six months of formal study each year, and in its Annual Announcement for 1892–93 noted that "while sound theoretical knowledge will be imparted, practical instruction will be the main feature of the college." This instruction included "free clinics . . . given twice a week, with a view to affording each student an opportunity to become familiar with the practical part of the profession."

The announcement also observed that "Students are expected to practice the greater part of the summer with a qualified practitioner," a requirement anticipating later intern and preceptorship programs.

Incidentally, the total cost of the college's two year course was $175, with good board available in Cincinnati for from $3 to $6 per week.

Ohio's second private veterinary college was established in Cincinnati four years after the first closed its doors. This was the Cincinnati Veterinary College, considered during its lifetime one of the better private schools. Considerably more successful than Ohio's first school, it remained in operation for two decades and graduated over 400 veterinarians. The college finally closed its doors in 1920 in the twilight of private veterinary education.

Both of these private schools made substantial contributions to veterinary medicine in Ohio; in graduating nearly 500 students, they helped meet the rapidly expanding need for trained practitioners. But despite this, they remained secondary influences, their private efforts overshadowed by public activity. Because in Ohio, the creative center of veterinary education was the Ohio State University.

And that brings us back to Dr. Norton Townshend.

When Ohio finally took advantage of the Morrill Land Grant Act eleven years after its passage, the result was *The Ohio Agricultural and Mechanical College* (later OSU), which opened its doors in Franklin County in 1873.

Dr. Norton Townshend was one of the founders and the new school's first Professor of Agriculture. Of more significance for veterinary medicine, he was also an influential backer of scientific veterinary education and, from the first, he used his power and prestige to insure its inclusion in the curriculum.

Townshend did not get everything he wanted right away. Veterinary education was included, but not as a separate department. Instead, the Board of Trustees established a Department of Zoology and Veterinary Science and appointed a zoologist, Dr. Albert H. Tuttle, as professor. Provision was also made for the

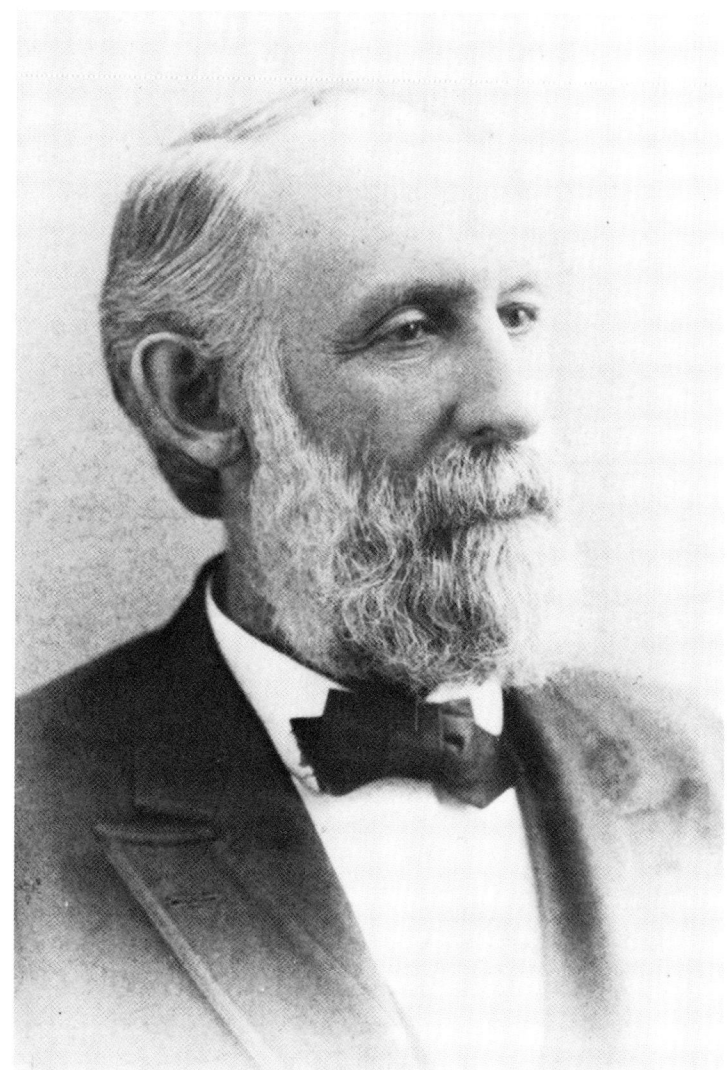

OSU President William H. Scott, 1893. He joined Professors Townshend and Tuttle in strongly advocating the creation of a separate chair of veterinary science at the University. In 1894, Dr. H. J. Detmers became the University's first Professor of Veterinary Medicine. (Photo Archives, Ohio State University)

teaching of some veterinary courses in the Department of Agriculture and Botany, with Dr. Townshend handling instruction pertaining to animal disease and its medical and surgical treatment.

It was a fragmented beginning for veterinary education but the Trustees of 1873 were guided by the realities of the period. Given the limited number of professional veterinarians, they recognized that it would be extremely difficult to attract enough qualified teachers for a separate department. Thus, the decision to divide responsibilities among two faculty members who, although not trained veterinarians, were well-acquainted with the discipline. And in Professors Townshend and Tuttle, they had men who would not remain satisfied with the "status quo."

Money was also a problem; Ohio's new A & M College had very little of it, a fact of which the Trustees were acutely aware. In their first Annual Report, they stressed the importance of veterinary medical training, but admitted that limited funding for "outfit and appliances" was impeding its development:

> In the department of zoology, the animal anatomy and physiology are now taught in a general way (no collections or illustrations) so that the foundation of a better knowledge of the animal economy is already laid, but this department also needs to be enlarged and extended, and thus veterinary science may be introduced and established on a sound basis with a very moderate additional expenditure, which as yet is beyond our means.

Eventually, the "moderate additional expenditure" was made and the Department of Zoology and Veterinary Science got its "outfit," including skeletons, alcohol-injected specimens, a life-size manikin and a full set of models illustrating the anatomy of man and the domestic animals. The acquisitions may seem meager by later standards, but Professor Tuttle was starting from scratch; he was enthusiastic and anticipated more progress:

> I trust that before the end of another year the institution will enjoy facilities for teaching the structure and functions of the body, second only to those possessed by medical colleges, and for reaching its relations in structure and function to the lower animals, superior to those possessed by the majority of such institutions.

So there was progress early on. If there was not yet a separate department, there was veterinary educa-

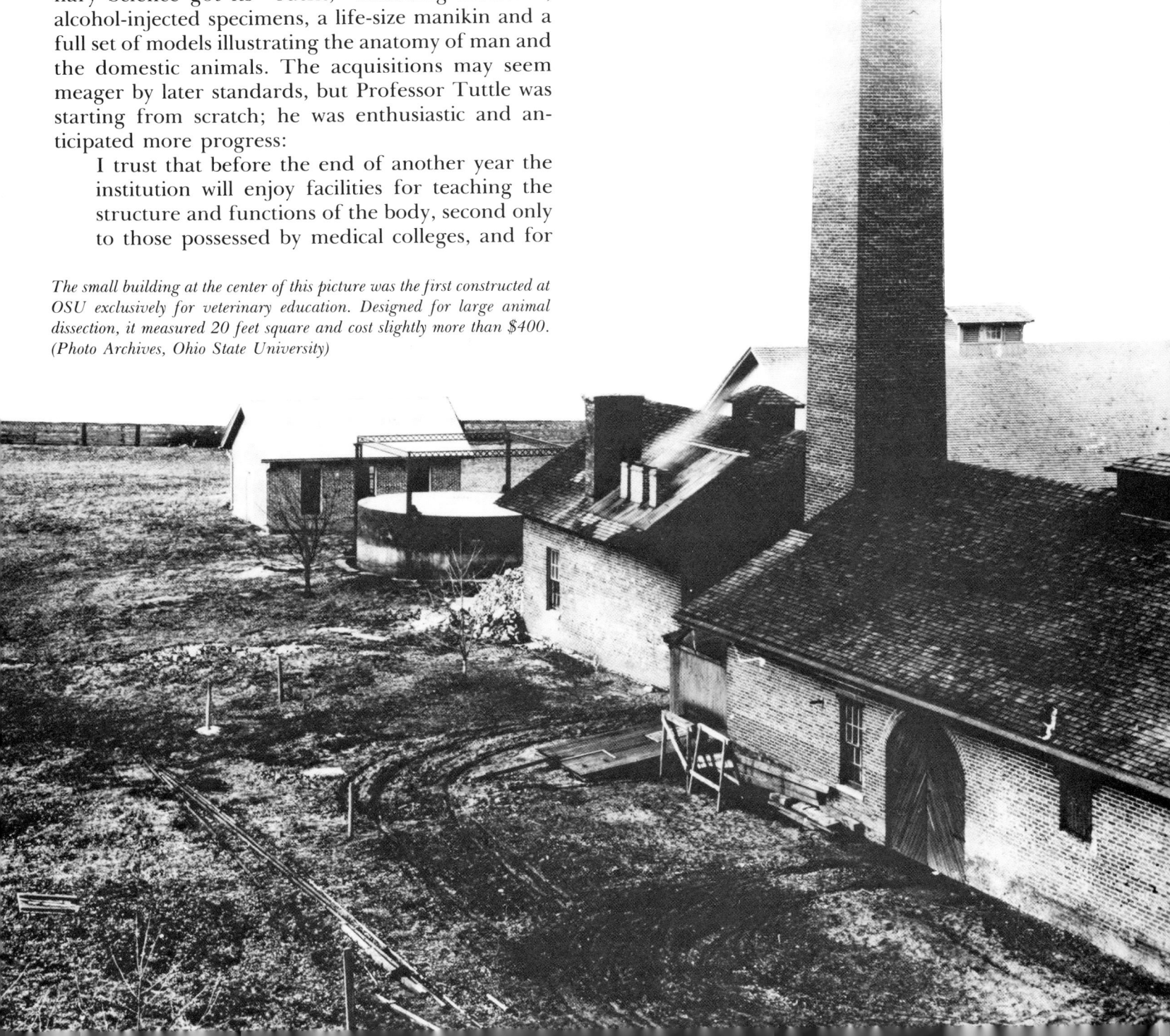

The small building at the center of this picture was the first constructed at OSU exclusively for veterinary education. Designed for large animal dissection, it measured 20 feet square and cost slightly more than $400. (Photo Archives, Ohio State University)

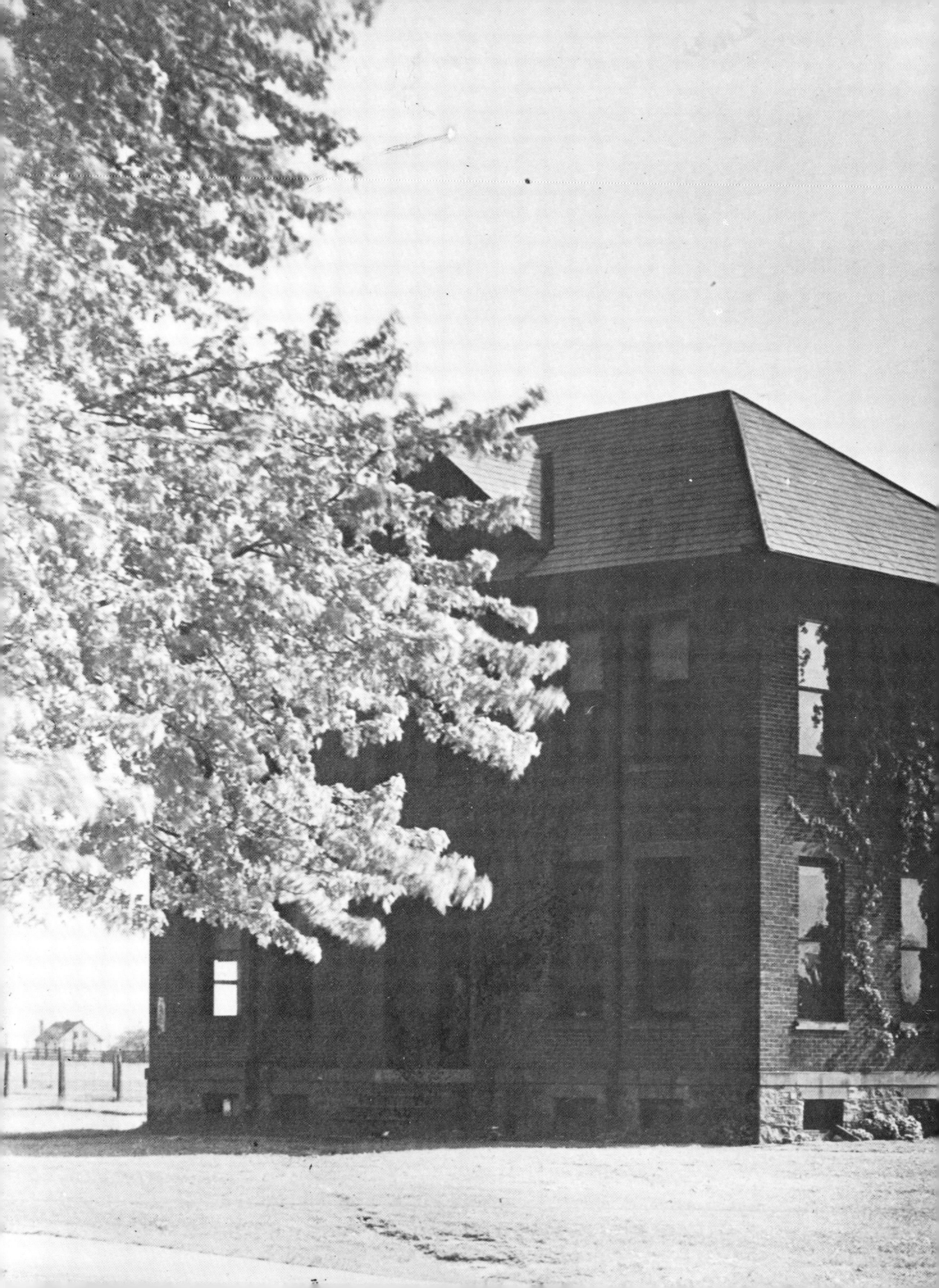

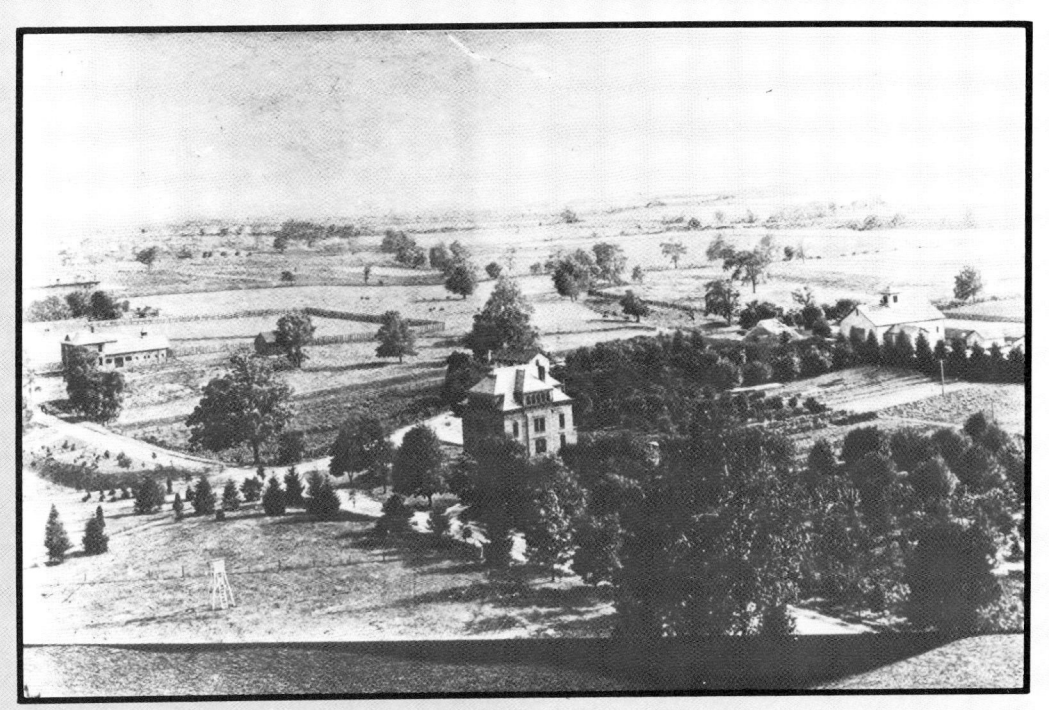

The Veterinary Hospital, first "home" of the OSU College of Veterinary Medicine. Completed in 1891, it remained in operation until 1910. The second photograph shows the Hospital in relation to the OSU campus.

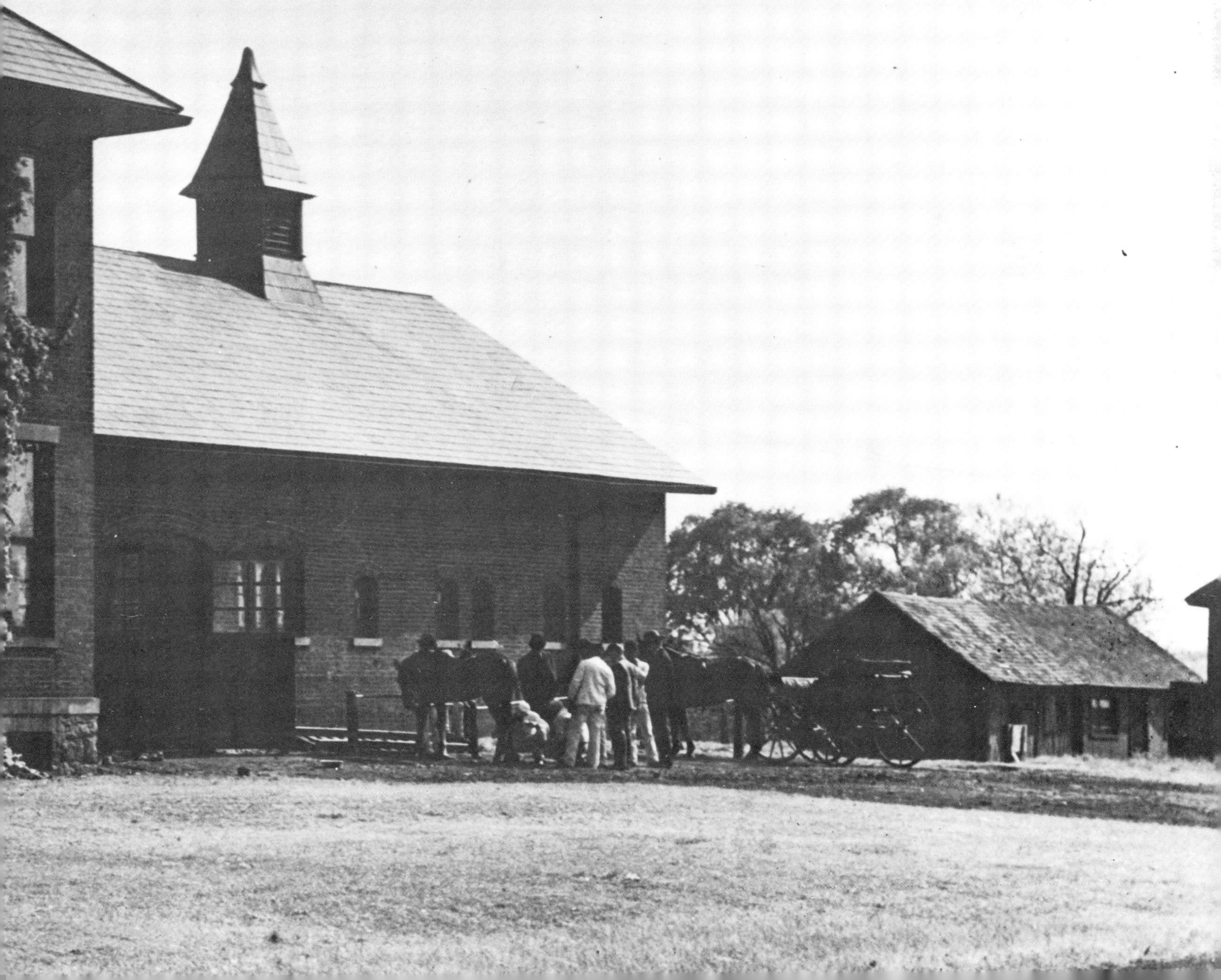

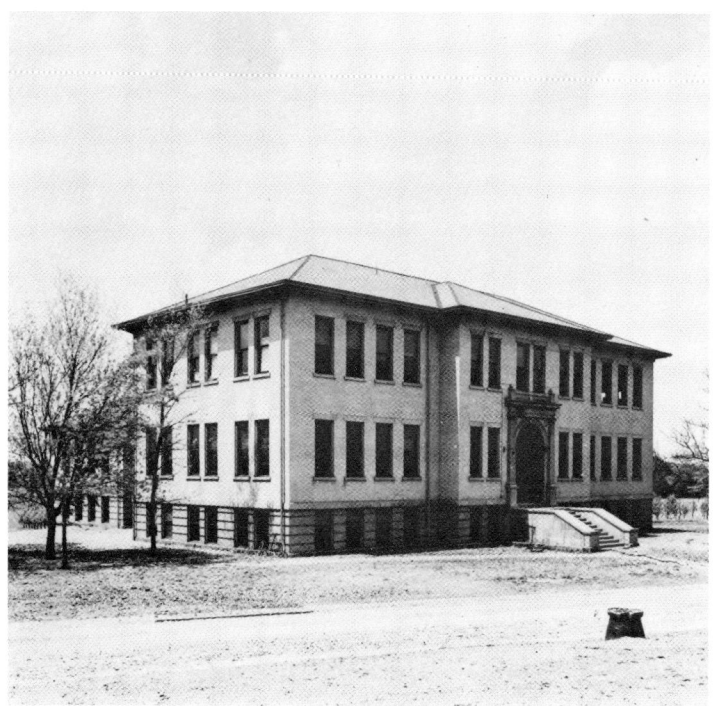

The Veterinary Laboratory. Constructed in 1903, it became the headquarters of the OSU College of Veterinary Medicine. (Photo Archives, Ohio State University)

tion. In November, 1875, Dr. Townshend, in his departmental report, wrote:

> Students of agriculture devoted the first term of the college year to the study of domestic animals, their varieties, special adaptations and management. The second term was occupied with the study of diseases to which domestic animals are subject; attention being particularly directed to the symptoms, causes, nature and prevention of disease, and to the action of medicine.... Through the third term, the diseases most frequently met with in Ohio were made the subject of study.

These courses were well-attended, testifying to a considerable interest in veterinary medicine. In his *History of the College of Veterinary Medicine,* Dr. Arthur F. Schalk notes that:

> ... Many students coming to the college from farms and recognizing the economic necessity of disease control took all of the veterinary courses in the agricultural curricula; sometimes their numbers equalled or exceeded those who chose the conventional agricultural courses.

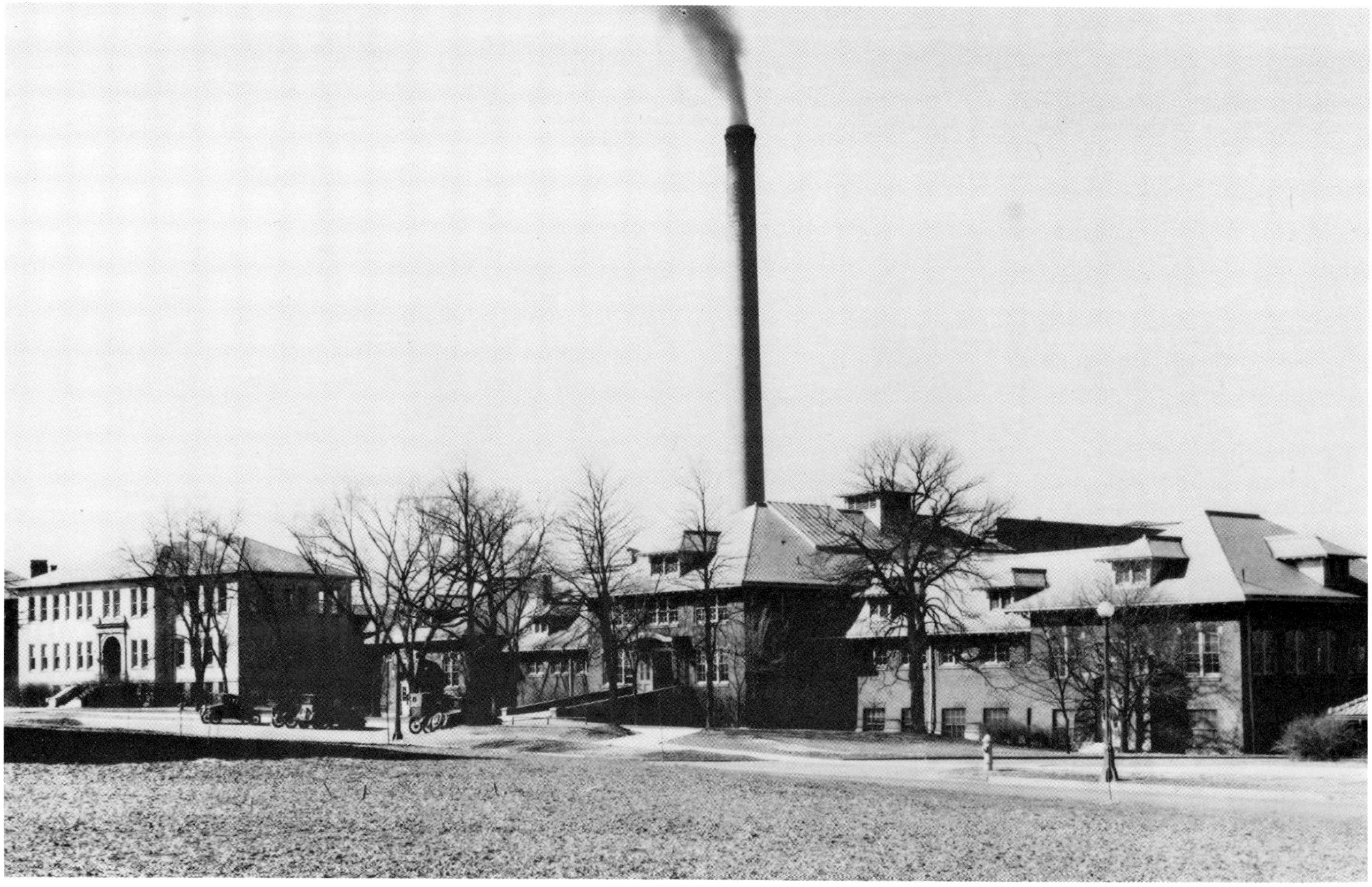

The Veterinary Clinic building, constructed in 1910 adjacent to the Veterinary Laboratory, was a major veterinary education facility at OSU until the 1950s. (Photo Archives, Ohio State University)

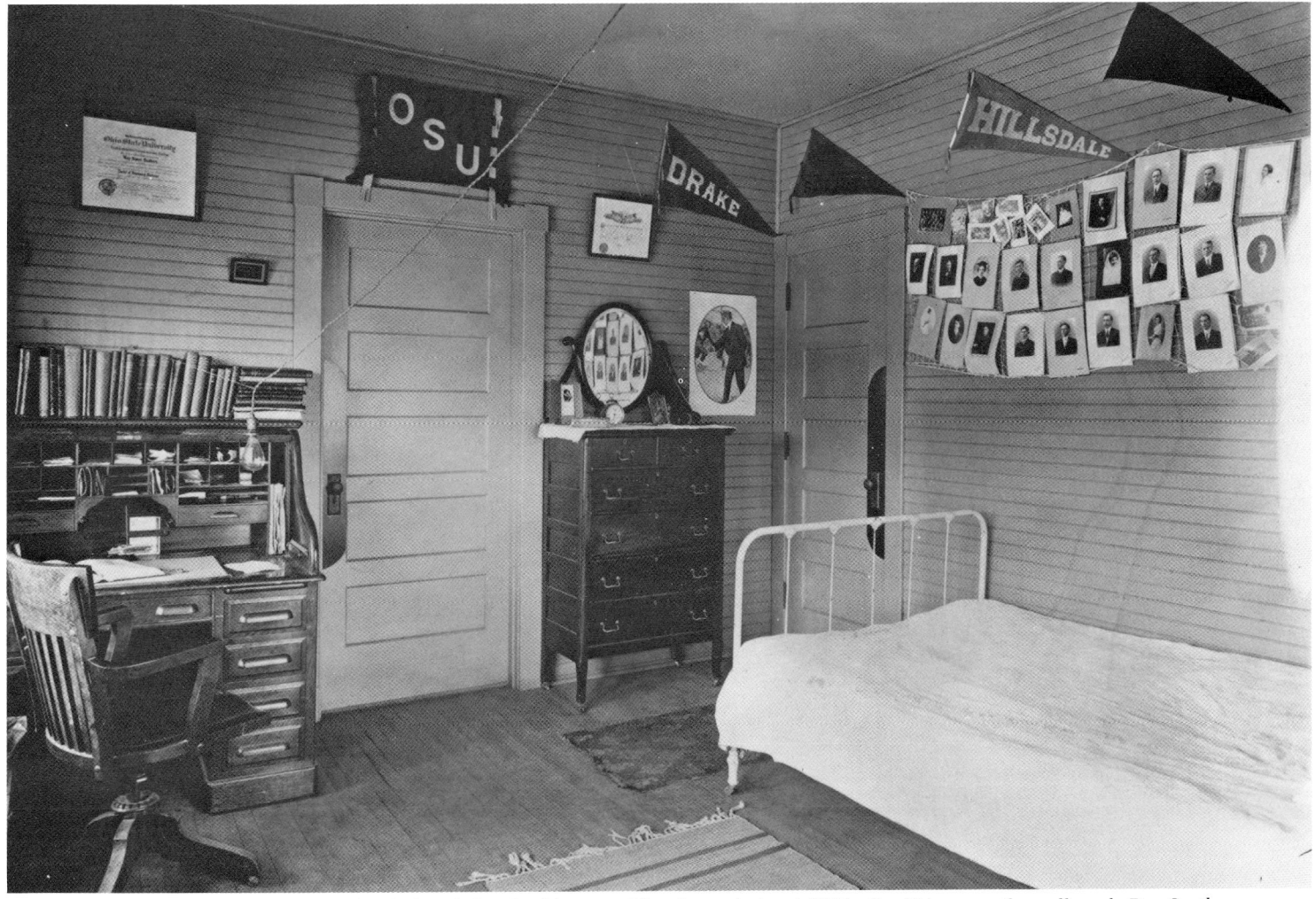
Interns on duty at the Veterinary Clinic worked and slept in this room. The picture is dated 1911; the diploma on the wall reads Ray Scothorn. (Photo Archives, Ohio State University)

This interest was paralleled by a growing public recognition of the importance of veterinary education. From the very first, livestock owners sought help from the new college and it was forthcoming. Dr. Townshend also noted this development in his 1875 report:

> Assistance from this department has in several instances been solicited by the owners of stock ... a disease of sheep ... which has prevailed in Licking County and in other parts of the state, was carefully investigated and found to depend on the presence of immense numbers of parasitic worms ... the natural history of the parasite was made public, together with an effective remedy against its ravages ... a troublesome and persistent cough affecting a number of cattle in the vicinity of Columbus ... was studied by examination of the affected animals after death ... the cough was found to be but a symptom of tubercular consumption, a disease that justifies all reasonable measure for its prevention, but does not very well reward any effort (with) a cure.... The hog cholera has also received attention and many animals, both living and dead, were inspected and valuable conclusions reached on points relating to the nature of the disease and its treatment.... Detailed statements ... have been published in the report of the State Board of Agriculture.... *It may not be out of place here to suggest that such investigations, if carefully and skillfully conducted, can scarcely fail to be of great advantage to the State.*

A year after Professor Townshend's report, veterinary education underwent its first departmental change; veterinary courses were removed from Zoology and consolidated in the Department of Agriculture, Botany and Veterinary Science. But this change did not satisfy either Professor Townshend or Professor Tuttle. Both men were aware of their limitations as veterinary teachers and for nearly a decade they continued to press for the establishment of a separate and distinct professorship of veterinary medicine. In 1883, they gained the strong support of the newly-formed OVMA, which also recognized the

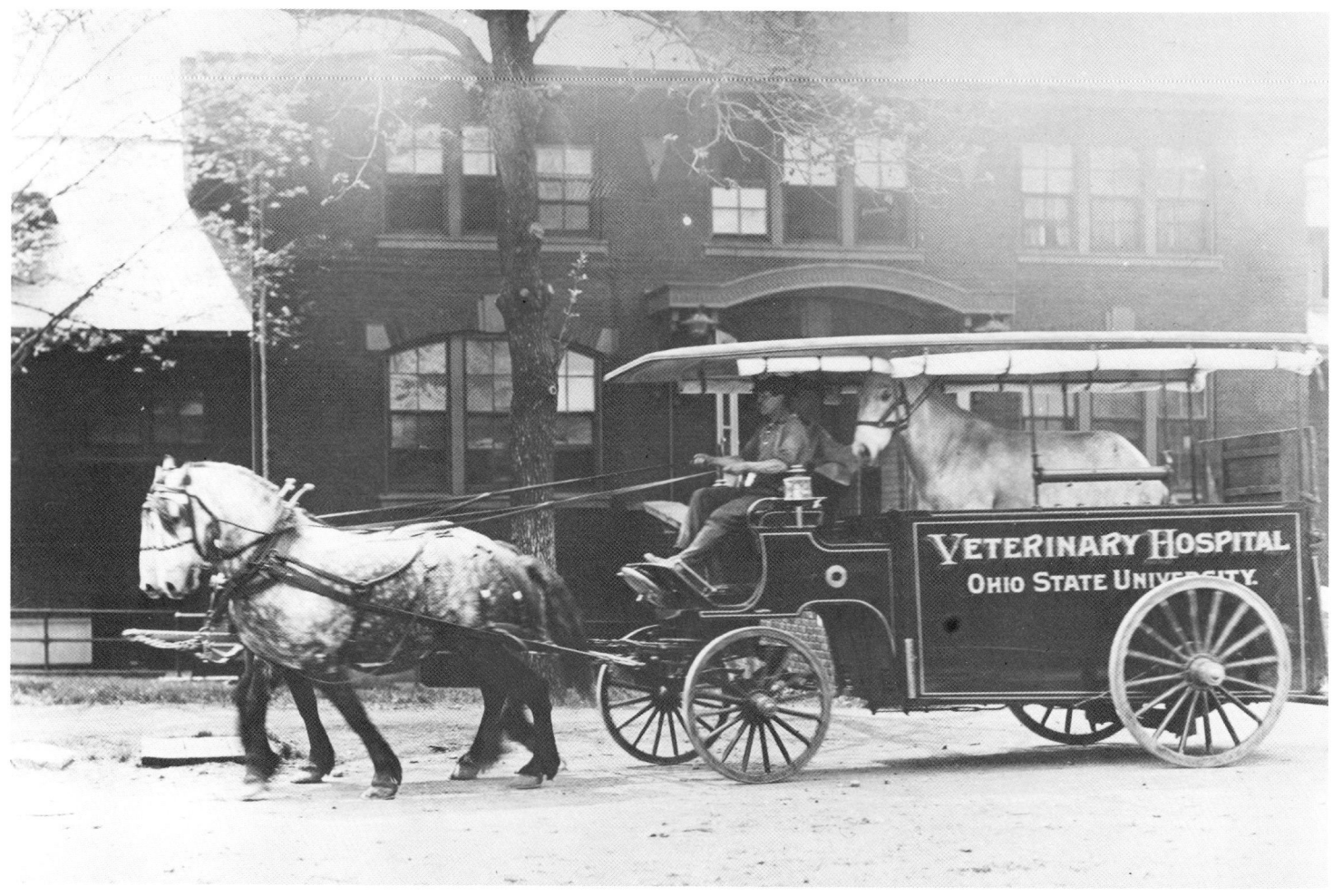

The Hospital's large animal ambulance, 1914. (Reprinted from The First Hundred Years: A Family Album of the Ohio State University, 1870-1970. *Copyright 1970 by the Ohio State University Press. All rights reserved)*

need for a trained veterinarian on the faculty. And, in January, 1884, *The Ohio Farmer* reported that OSU President Dr. William Scott had joined the campaign. Reporting on the 39th annual Agricultural Convention of Ohio, the *Farmer* wrote:

> By request Prof. Townshend explained the course of study for young farmers at the University. Dr. Scott, the President of the University, followed with an address, ably presenting its claims upon the agriculturists of the State. He showed the desirability of adding to the present faculty a chair of agricultural chemistry and of veterinary science.

Dr. Scott also urged farmers to contact their legislative representatives to support "these and other University needs." If they did, then it is entirely possible that grass-roots lobbying tipped the scales, for the same year the Board of Trustees gave veterinary education in Ohio its biggest boost to date. They established a professorship of veterinary surgery in the Department of Agriculture, Botany and Veterinary Science and to fill it picked a veterinarian named H.J. Detmers.

(Past records assign Professor Detmers a variety of first names: Heinrich, Henrich, Hinrich and Henry. To avoid compounding the uncertainty, we will call him "H.J. Detmers.")

The next year, 1885, even before Professor Detmers began teaching, the Trustees also established the OSU *School* of Veterinary Medicine, but this seemed to have no immediate significance. For several years, Detmers himself would refer to veterinary medicine as a "department" even though, in 1889, he was officially designated "Chief of the School." However, as Dr. Schalk observes, this latter action indicates that "the Board at least accepted the organization of Veterinary Medicine as an independent school notwithstanding many indications to the contrary."

The first veterinarian on the OSU faculty had a broad background in veterinary medicine. A graduate of the Royal Veterinary College in Berlin, H.J. Detmers emigrated to the United States in 1865 and was during his pre-Ohio career a private practitioner, teacher at several universities and a government veterinarian. At the time of his OSU appointment, he was a special agent in infectious diseases with the U.S. Department of Agriculture.

Detmers has been described as a man of unusual qualifications and capabilities who was "about a quarter of a century ahead of the time." He confirmed this almost immediately; the first thing Detmers wanted at OSU was a four-year course of veterinary study, something literally unheard of in the period. It was an ambitious proposal, but as Dr. Schalk notes "the time for such extensive training was not at hand."

The fact is, students stayed away in droves, choosing instead the two and three-year courses offered by other institutions rather than OSU's four-year challenge. Detmers had to be satisfied with something less, a three-year course which he vigorously defended as essential for the continued progress of the profession:

> I take it to be our object to give thorough instruction, and to send out veterinarians who shall fully deserve the confidence of the people. This cannot be done in a shorter time than is required by our course; neither can such studies as chemistry, botany, histology, laws of hygiene, microscopy, etc., be dispensed with in the present age. The time when a veterinarian could get along without them fortunately belongs to the past.... We (OSU) must, at least, be satisfied with quality rather than quantity, and cannot expect a large number of students.

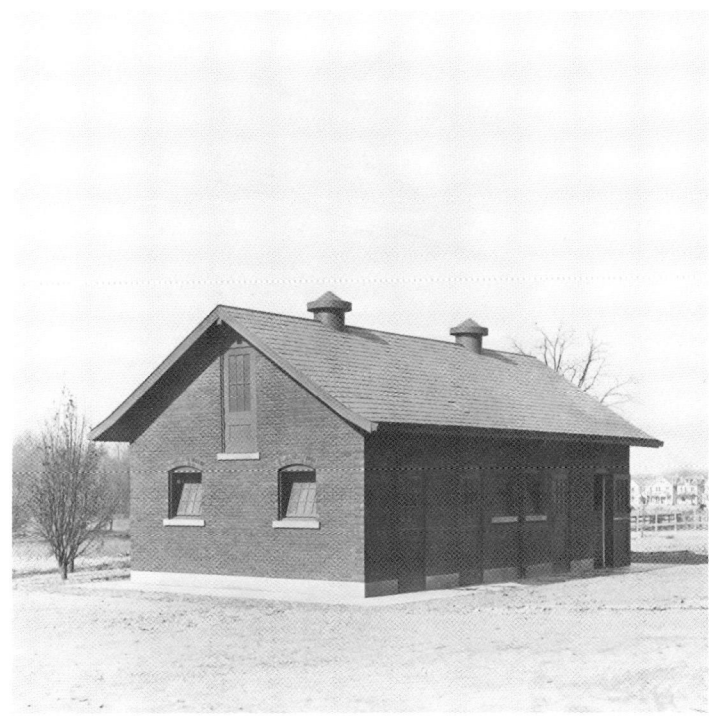

This eight-stall isolation ward was built in 1910, the same year as the Veterinary Clinic. Nearly a half century would pass before the Veterinary College gained another new building. (Department of Photography, Ohio State University)

Ambulance service as well as care was provided by the OSU Veterinary Hospital. This was the small animal ambulance in 1910. (Photo Archives, Ohio State University)

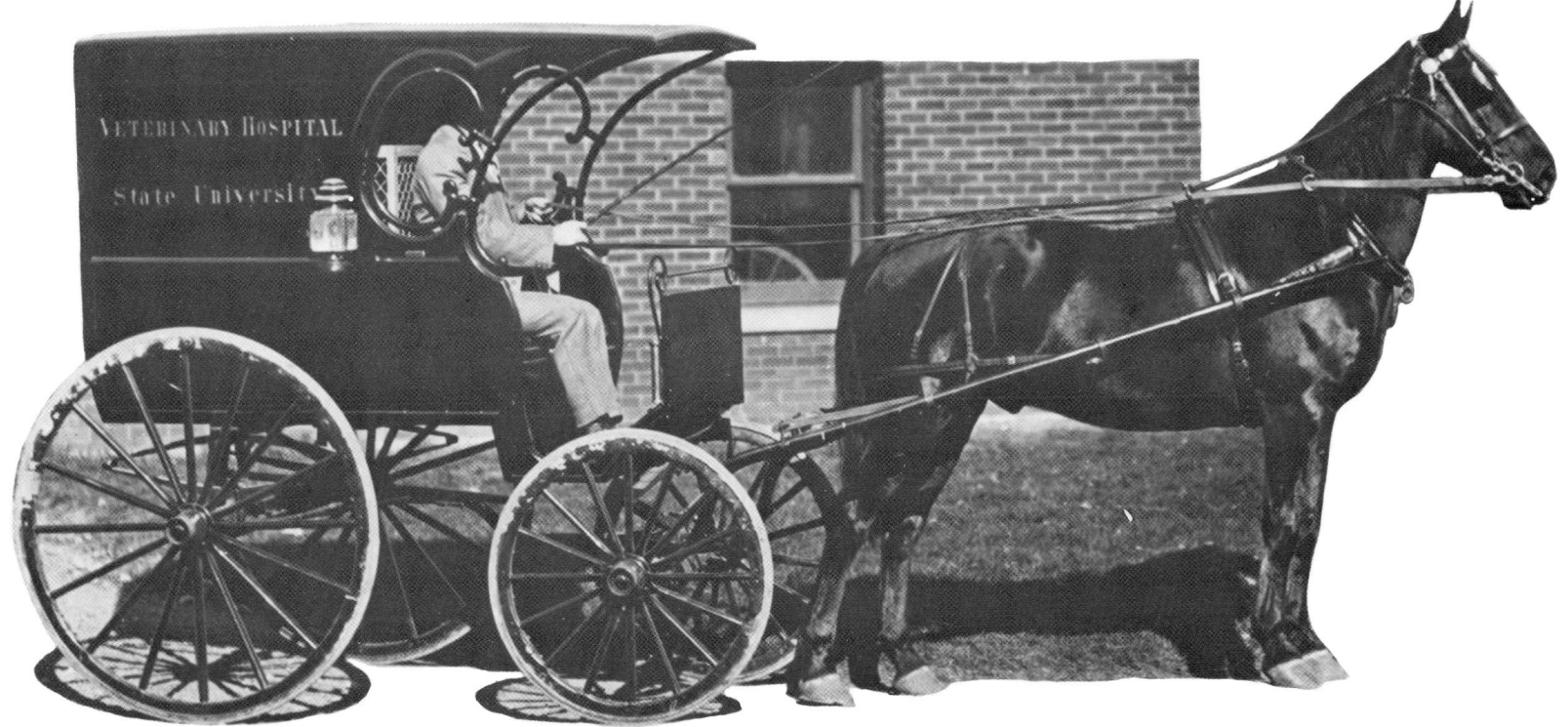

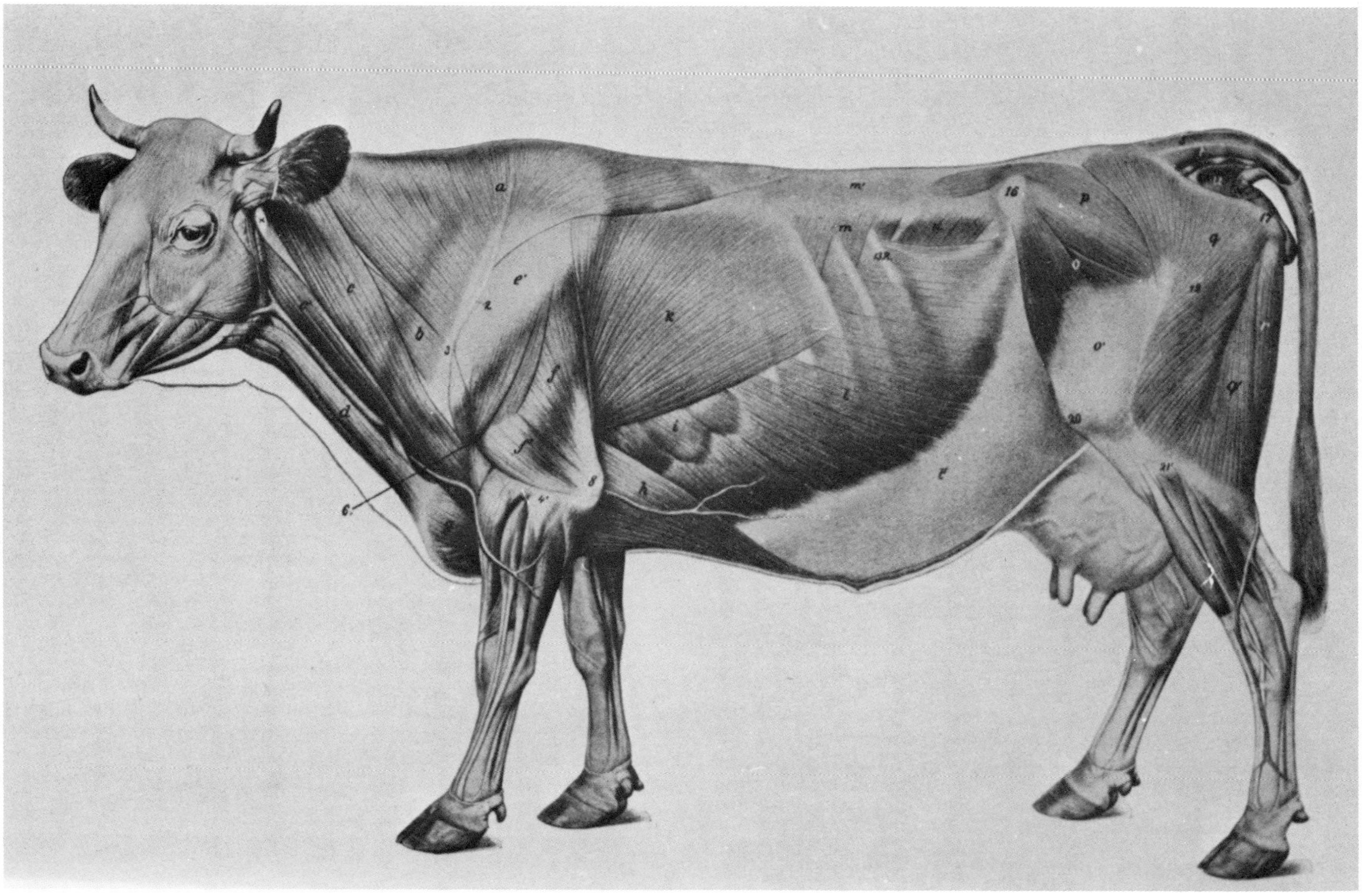

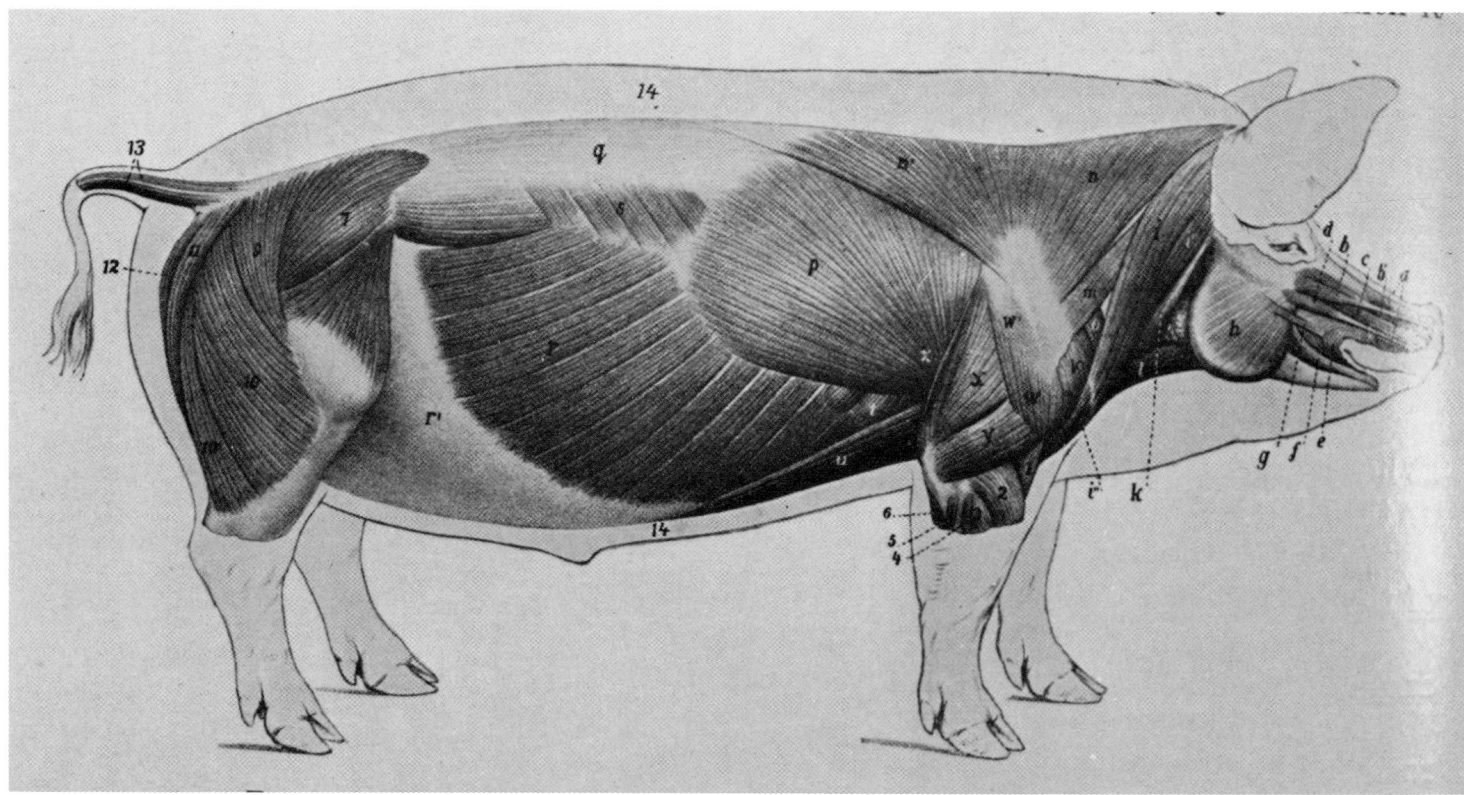

Two illustrations from the 1914 edition of Professor Septimus Sisson's The Anatomy of Domestic Animals, *a textbook so accurate and comprehensive that it is still in use today. (Ohio Historical Society)*

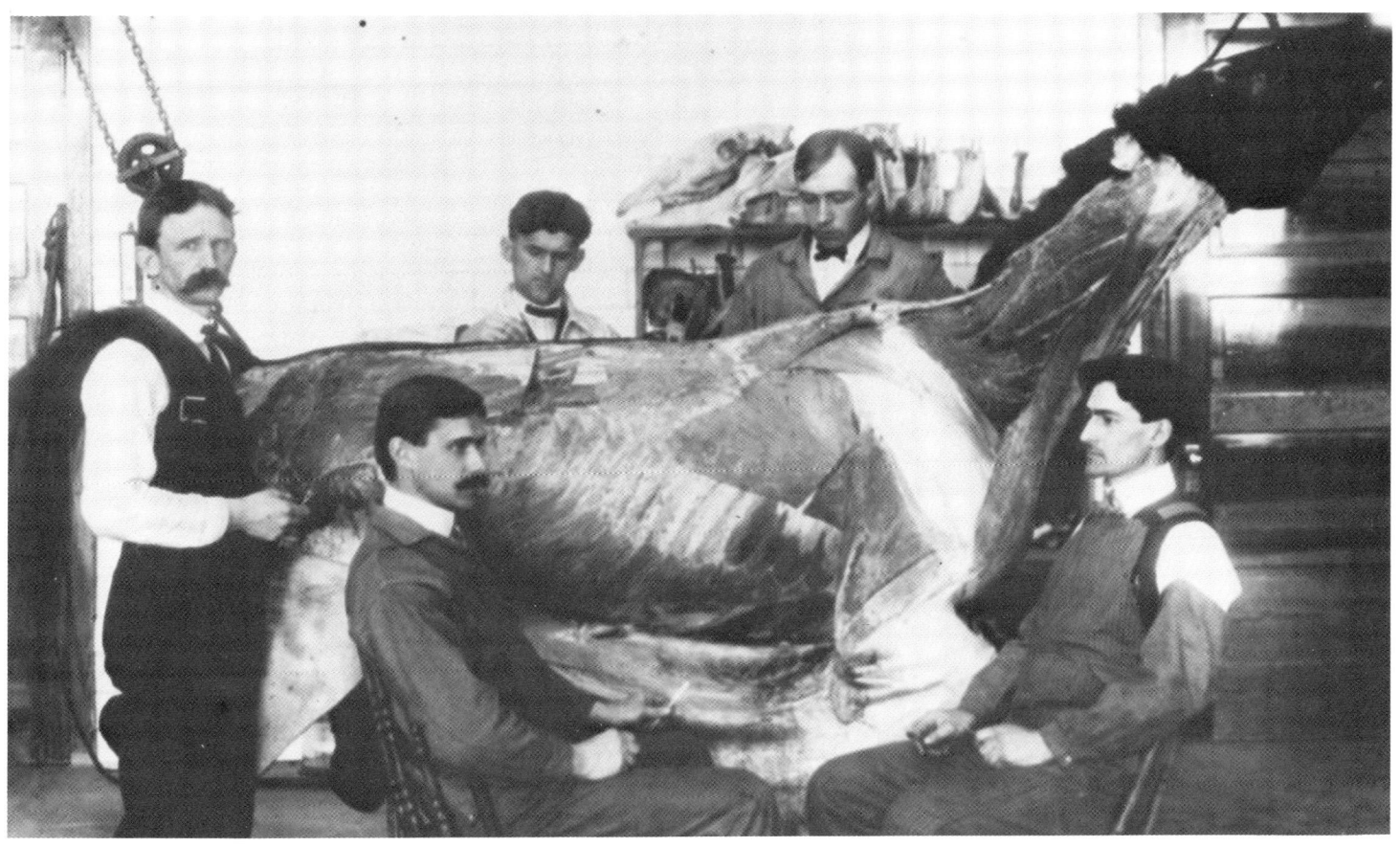

The OSU Veterinary Medicine Dissection Room, 1909. (Reprinted from The First Hundred Years: A Family Album of the Ohio State University, 1870-1970. *Copyright 1970 by the Ohio State University Press. All rights reserved)*

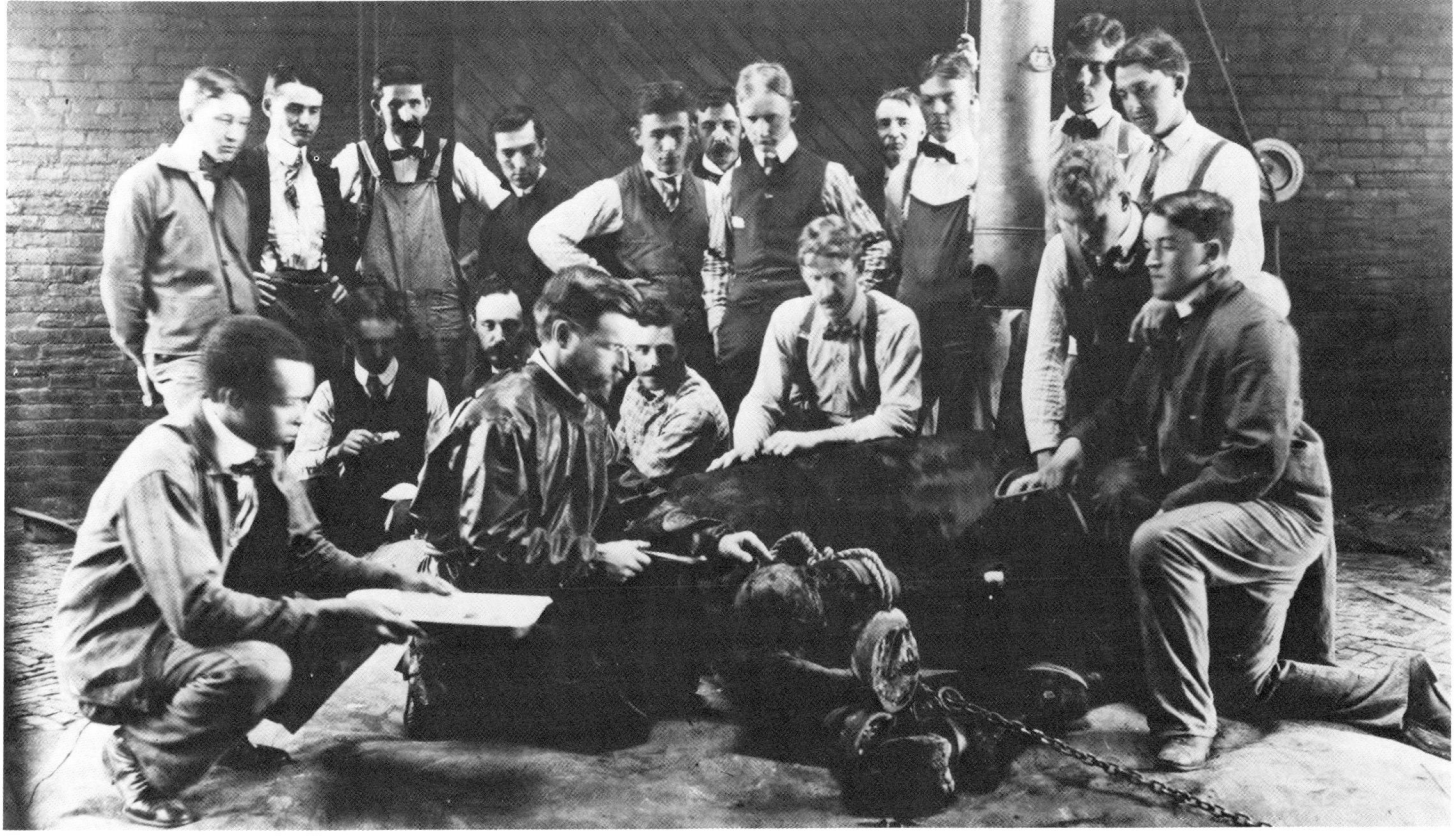

Veterinary students observe live surgery by Dean David White in 1897. White succeeded Professor Detmers as head of the OSU Veterinary College. (Photo Archives, Ohio State University)

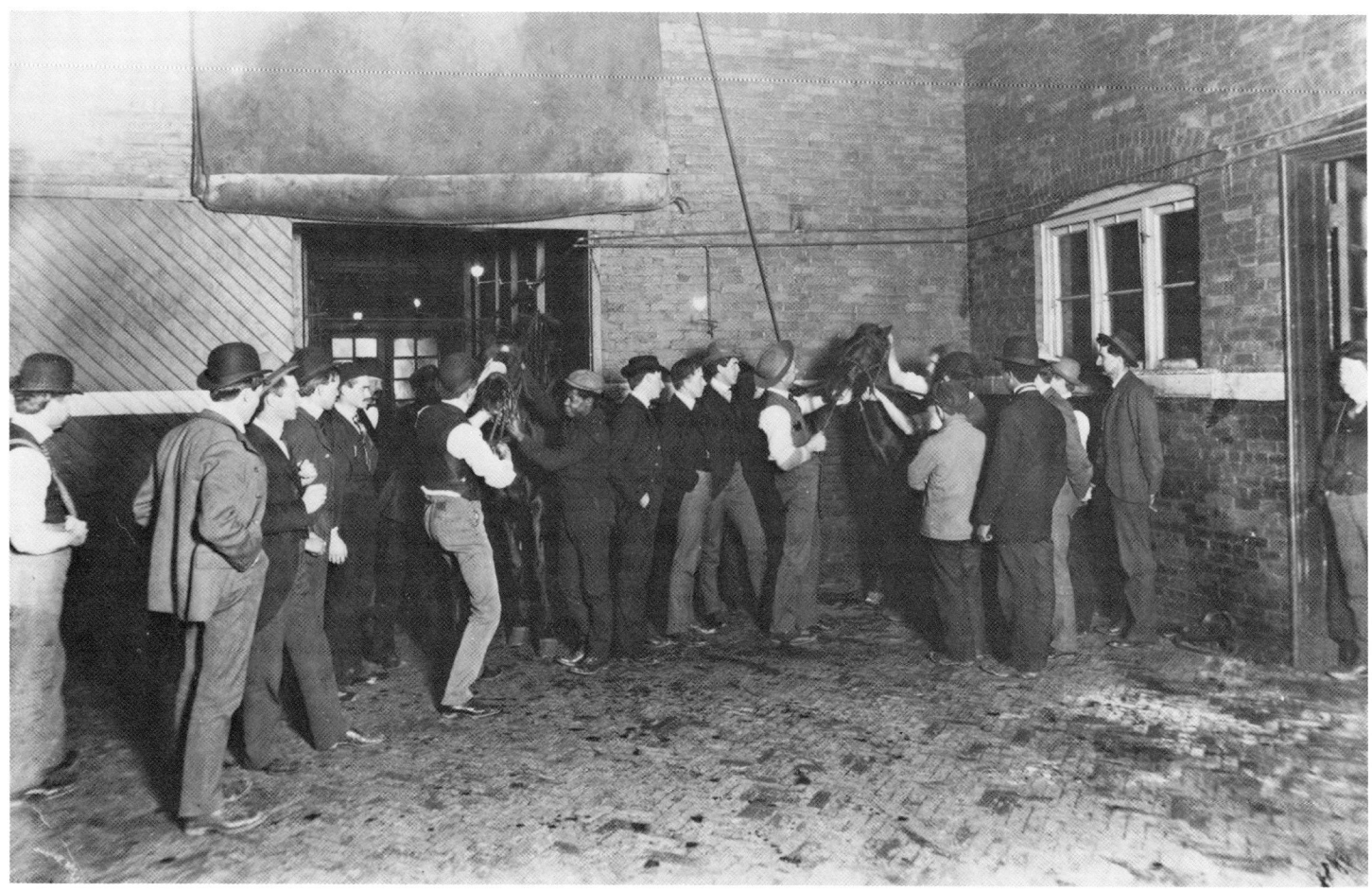
Veterinary students at a class in 1895. The dress code seems to have been somewhat stricter in those days. (Photo Archives, Ohio State University)

Detmers was right. In this period there was no large quantity of students; he reported classes of 3 to 5. But there was quality and in addition to the studies cited above, Detmers pioneered with other courses. Again, quoting Dr. Schalk:

> Helminthology and bacteriology were sciences that were in their very infancy in the last quarter of the 19th Century. Dr. Detmers organized a class in the former in 1886 and one in the latter in 1887.... Insofar as we can determine, these courses in bacteriology were the first that were projected in veterinary curricula in America...

Detmers was also strongly research-oriented, both in his work at OSU and in related activity at the Ohio Agricultural Experiment Station, where for a time he was a staff member. In 1886, in the first annual report of the Veterinary Science Department (or School), he wrote:

> I have since August, not only answered several inquiries in regard to diseases of animals, but also undertaken experiments for the purpose of ascertaining the true cause or causes of some infectious diseases, with a view of devising rational and effective means of prevention. The principal line of experiments, commenced in August, were undertaken for the purpose of ascertaining the real cause of swine-plague or so-called hog-cholera.

And five years later, in another annual summary, Detmers reported:

> In bacteriology some work has been done which, I am sure, will prove to be of more than temporary interest. Already, last year.... I succeeded in devising means to prevent swine-plague by a protective inoculation.

Detmers retired from OSU in 1895, returning to private practice and research. He left behind a rich legacy: ten years of leadership that had taken scientific veterinary education in Ohio from an embryonic beginning to a position of national prominence. Recognizing that quality education and research were crucial to the profession and those it served, he championed both, setting standards and precedents that would guide his successors in the decades to come.

The years immediately following Detmer's retirement were marked by a growing demand for even broader and more scientific veterinary training, a trend that confirmed his influence. It was an effort in which the OVMA was prominently involved; the Association and its members were vocal exponents of

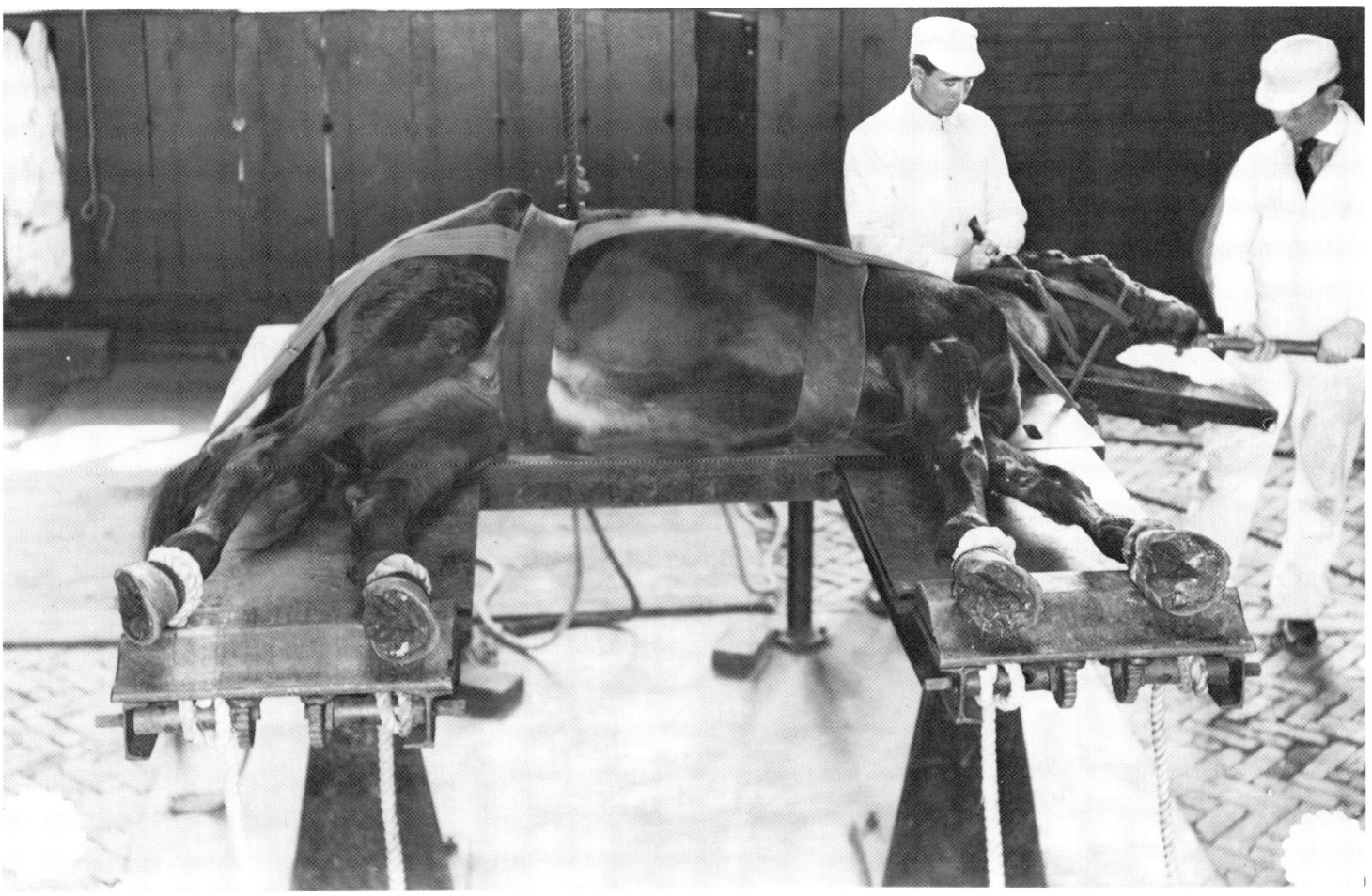
A horse is readied for surgery by veterinary students in 1912. (Photo Archives, Ohio State University)

higher standards and expanded studies at what had become, in 1895, the College of Veterinary Medicine. Progress did not come overnight, but in 1915 Dr. Detmers' initial dream was finally realized. In a report to the OVMA Annual Meeting of 1915-16, the Committee on Legislation observed:

> It is a pleasure for us all to learn that the Veterinary College of the Ohio State University has adopted a four-year course and that the entrance requirements have been raised to a full high school course. (Specifically *first class* high school training or its equivalent.)

The committee cited the support roles of both the OVMA and the AVMA and also commended OSU for "the great desire of Ohios insitution to fulfill the promise of education and make the individual man more competent, more efficient to serve the public.

In this same period, the OVMA also supported the development of adequate physical facilities for the Veterinary College. These facilities were badly needed; in the first decade there had been no excessive spending on bricks and mortar. In fact, there had been none at all.

The first veterinary courses (and all other courses) were taught in University Hall, better known as "Old Main," which was the University's first and, for a time, only building. Here Professors Townshend and Tuttle carried on their lectures, demonstrations and laboratory work. In succeeding years other facilities were used; Dr. Detmers taught for a period in the Chemistry Building and, when it burned down in 1889, moved to the Agricultural Experiment Station building on Neil Avenue.

It was not until 1886, three years after the founding of the OVMA, that a building was constructed specifically for veterinary education purposes. It was a small beginning, a 20 foot square structure for large animal dissection. The Board of Trustees noted the expenditure in their Annual Report:

> The house for dissecting purposes has been constructed at a cost of $417.25 and a model horse has been ordered which will cost about $900.

The money came from a $2,000 legislative appropriation for veterinary education. This, incidentally, was the first appropriation of any kind for OSU since it opened its doors as Ohio A & M in 1873.

Construction of the dissecting "house" was a short first step. But four years later the Ohio General Assembly was more generous. Responding to the

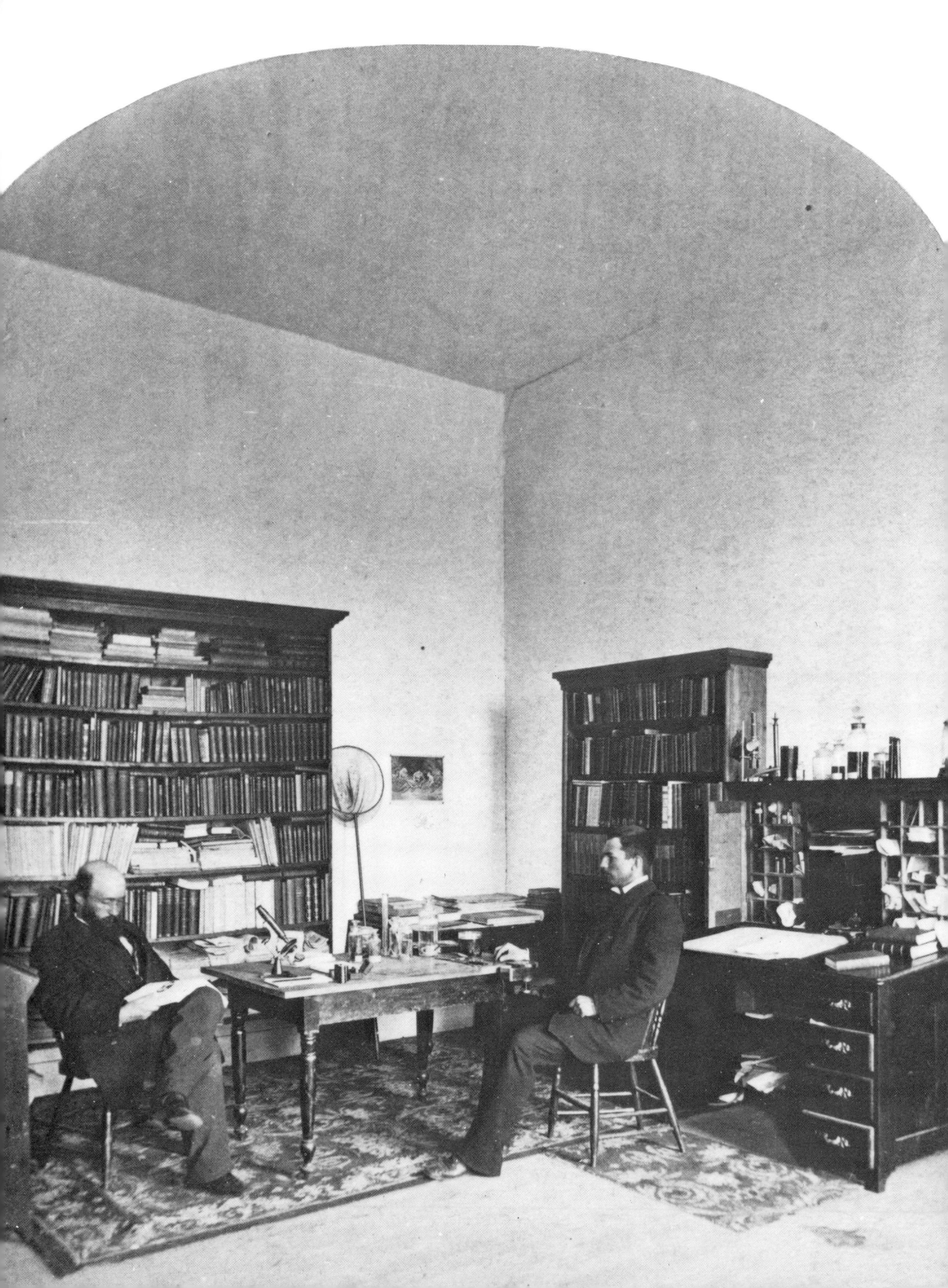

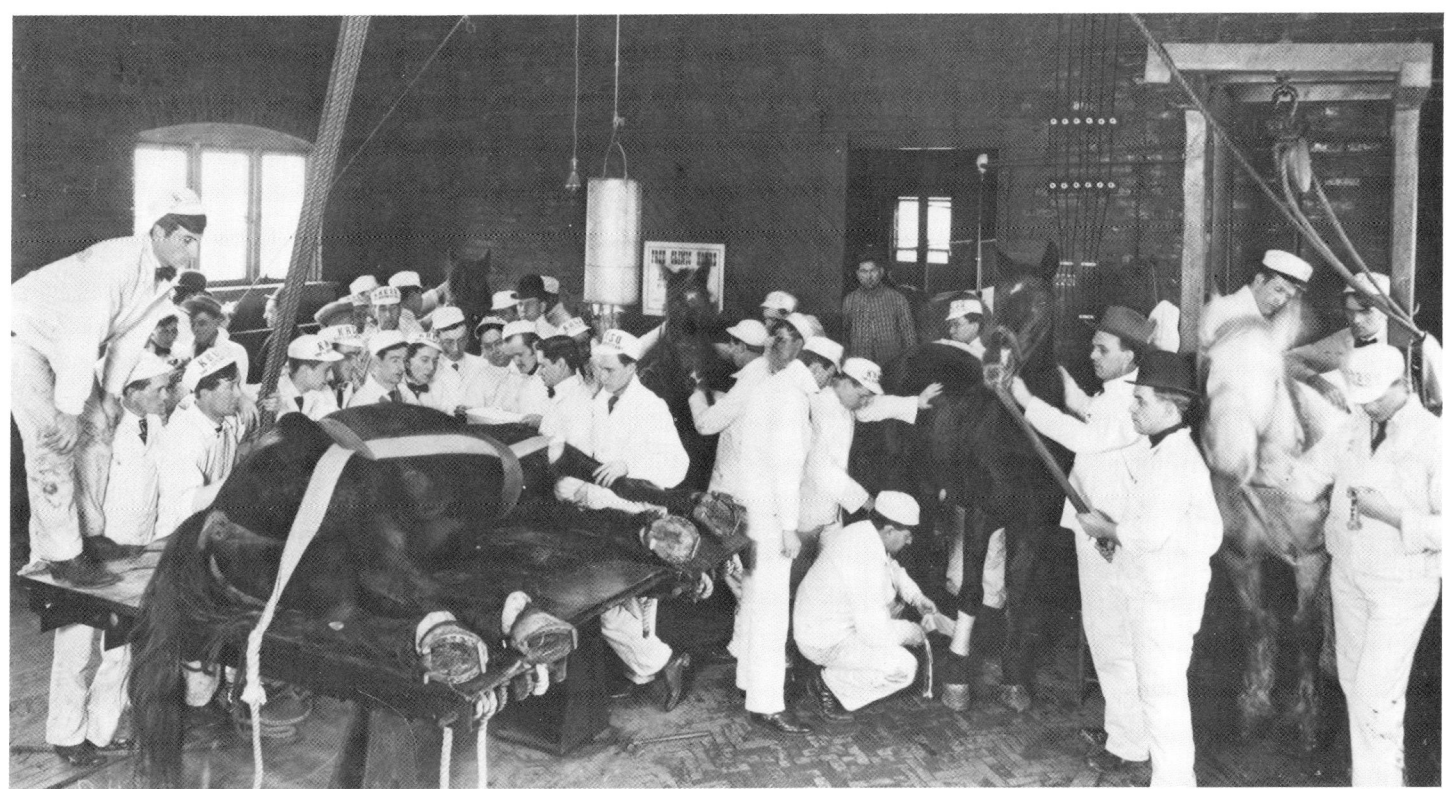

A 1915 class at the OSU Veterinary College. Equine care was still a major concern, a reflection of the continued importance of the horse. (Photo Archives, Ohio State University)

pleas of Dr. Detmers and others for a separate veterinary medicine building, the legislature in 1890 appropriated $5,000 "for a veterinary hospital, with accommodations for classes in such department." The College of Veterinary Medicine finally had a home of its own.

The new hospital, completed the following year, was impressive for the period; a contemporary report offers this description:

> The main part contains a basement for storage and the furnace, and in the 1st and 2nd stories a museum, drug store, office and sleeping room for the use of students attending patients in the hospital, a lecture room and office for the professor in charge, a room for experiments in bacteriology, a photographic dark room and ample halls . . . the rear part contains a clinic room 28 × 30 for the examination of patients and for surgical operations. The remainder of this portion of the building is occupied by a stable 28 × 31 where animals will be cared for under treatment.

The same year the Veterinary College also gained two additional structures, a new large animal dissection building and, adjacent to it, a small temporary barn used as an isolation ward and postmortem room for large animals.

For the next 12 years, the Hospital remained the center of veterinary education activity. But in 1903 it lost its primacy; the new $37,000 Veterinary Laboratory was completed and became the headquarters of the College of Veterinary Medicine. And, in 1910, the Hospital ceased operation, replaced by a new Veterinary Clinic Building, erected at the then impressive cost of $130,000. The same year, an eight-stall isolation ward was built for animals with infectious and contagious diseases.

So, after an initial ten years of neglect, veterinary education gradually acquired an adequate physical plant. But while the period between 1890 and 1910 produced a sizable crop of buildings, it was succeeded by a drought of almost 50 years' duration. It would be the mid-1950s before the College of Veterinary Medicine saw another new structure.

More about that and other Veterinary College activities, including the OSU/OVMA connection, in succeeding chapters.

Professor Albert H. Tuttle, on the left, in his office at University Hall in 1876. A zoologist, Professor Tuttle headed the Department of Zoology and Veterinary Science. (Reprinted from The First Hundred Years: A Family Album of the Ohio State University, 1870–1970. *Copyright 1970 by the Ohio State University Press. All rights reserved)*

The Ohio Farmer

Devoted to the Improvement and Betterment of the Farmer, His Family and Farm

The Control of Bovine Tuberculosis
Some Notes on Experience with this Great Dairy Scourge

By C. C. Hayden,
Ohio Experiment Station

From the financial standpoint tuberculosis is the second most menacing disease affecting dairy cattle, abortion probably standing first in losses caused. So much has been written for and against the possibility of eradicating this disease from dairy herds that the subject has become somewhat callous to the minds of many dairymen. They are not fully convinced that it is possible for the ordinary dairyman to clean up his herd and, therefore, are inclined to do the ostrich stunt and close their eyes to the signs of danger. Meanwhile the disease is at work and their lethargy gives it its chance to increase. Some are ignorant; some are doubtful as to the harm caused by the disease to both cattle and man; others are informed but do not care, if they can "get by" without the public finding out that their herds are diseased. Were most owners adequately aware of many disastrous experiences they might take warning.

The widespread agitation by consumers and breeders against the disease will not cease but will continue until some means of relief is found and the men who continue to "sleep" on the subject will be hardest hit when their cleaning up time comes.

"Line upon line and precept upon precept" is a good thing when such a sneaking, treacherous enemy is the subject. The germs of this disease are as stealthy and as treacherous as German spies. For many years they have been establishing themselves in our dairy herds where they are secretly eating out the vitality and vitals of our dairy animals. Once they are introduced into the body of a cow they set up a colony or center of infection from which the germs may be thrown off and other animals infected.

Often a single apparently healthy animal has been bought and placed in a herd where she has infected, directly or indirectly, from 10 to 90 percent of the herd. The owner is greatly surprised and sorely tried when, all too late, he learns what damage has been done. Too great care can not be taken to keep diseased animals away from the healthy herd. The writer has in mind a herd where a cow was introduced for a short time to be bred to the herd sire. The result was the infection of several other members of the herd, causing great loss. No man is safe in introducing an animal into his herd without it be quarantined and carefully tested; and even then he is not absolutely safe if the animal is mature. There are other avenues thru which a herd may become infected.

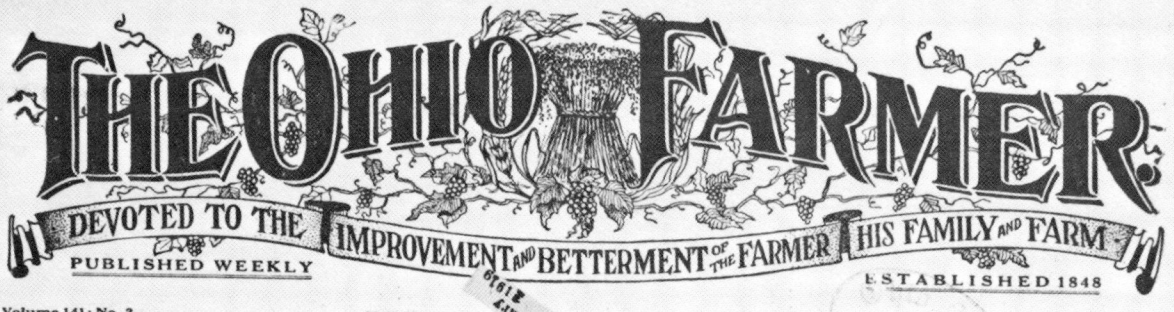
"IT TAKES CONSIDERABLE COURAGE TO MAKE UP ONE'S MIND TO TEST A GOOD HERD OF PUREBREDS."

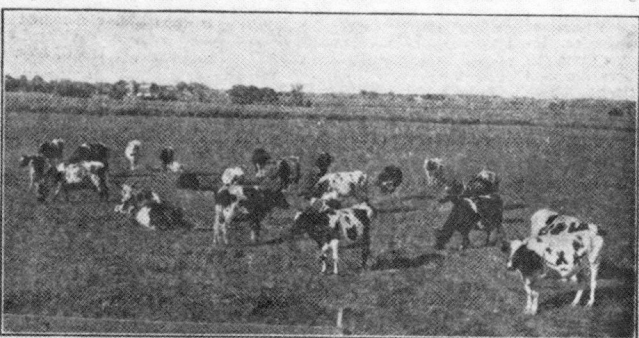
AN ALL-CONCRETE DAIRY ESTABLISHMENT—FIREPROOF AND EASILY DISINFECTED.

It is possible that the infection may come from cattle in an adjoining pasture by licking each other thru the fence. In sections where there are creameries, it is spread by feeding unpasteurized skimmilk from the creameries. There is always danger in placing healthy cattle in a barn where other cattle have been kept, unless the barn has been cleaned and disinfected.

In most cases the disease develops so secretly and so slowly that it is not suspected until a test is made or the animal is nearly gone. In many herds it exists for years without being detected, where no tests are made, and many owners who are aware of its presence try to keep it a secret, fearing the financial loss which may follow a test. The careful buyer is well aware how "cock-sure" the man is who never tests his herd, that his cows are healthy, and how difficult it is to get men to admit that their herds are not free from the disease. Justice in this matter requires that men deceive neither themselves nor their neighbors.

When one or more animals become so infected that they are throwing off the germs from the lungs or bowels or both, the remainder of the herd will become infected rapidly, tho it may not become outwardly visible for many years. Animals may die of the disease and the cause not be suspected unless a post-mortem examination is made. Unlike the majority of serious diseases, if the animal is well fed, it does not seriously affect the vital functions nor even reduce greatly its flesh until well established thru the body or some vital organ is partly destroyed. The germs may never escape from the animal's body to infect others and the animal may recover; but one can not tell which is going to be the outcome. Therefore, a diseased or suspicious animal is always dangerous.

The detective with his thermometers, syringe and bottle of tuberculin can easily discover its presence in a herd and he is the only one who can detect it in the individual with any degree of certainty. If he is an expert, few cases will "get by" and such cases are those in which the germs have recently been taken into the body but have not begun to multiply, are dormant or in which the disease has advanced to such a stage that the animal becomes immune to the effects of tuberculin. The latter are the most dangerous cases but many of them can be detected by a careful external examination.

Is There a Way Out?

Well, what are dairymen to do about it anyway? The man who has a large herd which has not been tested is frightened when it is mentioned, if he is awake to the seriousness of the disease.

(Concluded on page 9.)

CHAPTER IV

ANIMAL DISEASE: THE GREAT CAMPAIGN

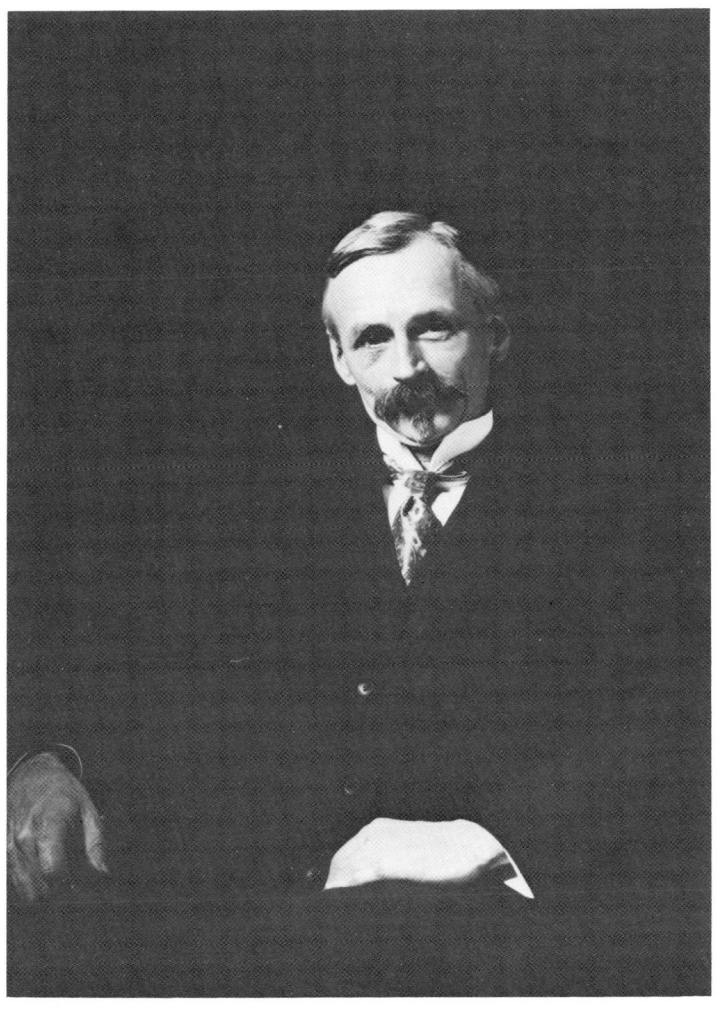

Dr. Septimus Sisson. One of the most distinguished members of the OSU Veterinary College faculty, he also was a leader in the OVMA, serving as Association president in 1914. (Photo Archives, Ohio State University)

Few men in Ohio had ever seen a case of this disease (foot-and-mouth). Like a bolt from the sky came this scourge upon the nation.

... about 45 percent of all the young men and boys from 15 to 30 years of age who die in Ohio are killed by tuberculosis, with milk the greatest source of infection.

As a farm youngster, I remember when farmers were just wiped out (by hog cholera) in the middle teens in southern Ohio. You could go along a county road and see hogs burning on both sides of the road. Almost a 100 percent mortality.

The Texas cattle fever has broken out among the cattle of certain sections of Clermont Co., Ohio . . . over one hundred head of cattle have already died and the disease is still spreading.

These quotes, all describing conditions in the early 1900s, sum up the greatest challenge then facing Ohio's newly-emerging veterinary profession. Animal disease was a grim and costly fact-of-life, and it was a menace not only to livestock but to the people who raised them and those who consumed their products.

Many diseases were chronic; they persisted year after year, a steady drain on resources, health, and life itself. Others erupted suddenly, as when a virulent epizootic of foot-and-mouth disease swept Ohio and a large part of the nation in 1914-15. Writing in *The American Veterinary Profession*, J.F. Smithcors described its *blitzkrieg* progress and the response:

The first appearance of the disease was . . . outside of Niles, Michigan, in August, 1914. By February 1915, 2,245 premises and 223 counties of 20 states and the District of Columbia had become infected. Since wholesale slaughter . . . was considered the best means of controlling contagious diseases, this was carried out on a large scale. Very rapidly, 68,776 cattle, 68,235 hogs and 9,087 sheep and goats were either slaughtered or died of the disease.

The Ohio Farmer, *January 19, 1918 (Ohio Historical Society)*

A CENTURY OF CARING

The Ohio Farmer, November 15, 1919 (Ohio Historical Society)

The Ohio Farmer, October 18, 1924 (Ohio Historical Society)

The Ohio Farmer, November 7, 1925 (Ohio Historical Society)

Headlines in The Ohio Farmer *chronicle the early years of Ohio's campaign against bovine tuberculosis. The eradication of this livestock scourge stands as one of the major achievements of veterinary medicine.*

In Ohio, some 12,000 head of livestock had to be destroyed at a dollar loss of some $400,000. And Ohio, which moved swiftly to destroy infected herds, had a comparatively low mortality rate.

Ironically, the outbreak of foot-and-mouth disease, costly as it was, had a beneficial impact on veterinary medicine. Smithcors says it "was largely instrumental for increased interest in the improvement of standards of veterinary education in the United States." And, at the height of the outbreak in Ohio, OVMA President, Dr. Septimus Sisson, told the Association's 1915 Annual Meeting:

> One of our greatest citizens said not long ago that the American people did not learn so much by experience as by calamities. It is probably true that the recent outbreak of foot-and-mouth disease, with the attendant serious financial losses and dislocation of trade, has done more to bring our profession before the public in a few weeks than all the previous half century of patient and unassuming service.

But if foot-and-mouth disease could be eliminated rather swiftly, there were other pervasive animal afflictions posing more formidable threats. Chief among these was bovine tuberculosis, a curse on both rural and urban America. For decades it would remain a stubborn adversary of the professional veterinarian.

At the turn of the century, tuberculosis was killing more people in the United States than any other disease; the death rate was close to 200 per 100,000 persons. Ten percent of human pulmonary tuberculosis and almost all other forms of human tuberculosis were of bovine origin, contracted from cattle, not other people.

The connection between sick cows and sick people was recognized, as the prevalence of the disease was not a matter of ignorance. But despite the warnings of professional veterinarians, the public remained largely indifferent. In 1889, at a meeting of the AVMA, Dr. Alexandre Liautard called for "some means of arousing public sentiment to the importance and grave dangers of this disease." Dr. Lachlan McLean suggested, "If milk cans from some of the herds infected with tuberculosis were labelled 'consumption at eight cents a quart' it would not be putting it too strong, and would probably arouse the people from their state of lethargy."

But the lethargy persisted for years and at all levels, including government. Ohio was no exception; in 1914, Dr. G. W. Cliffe told the OVMA Annual Meeting:

> We find that no state east of the Mississippi and north of the Mason-Dixon Line enjoys such lax

> ## THE OHIO FARMER
> # Declare War On Tuberculosis In Ohio
> ### Area Testing To Be Pushed So That More Cattle Owners Will Benefit
> #### By L. L. RUMMELL
>
> TUBERCULOSIS eradication in Ohio in the future will be on a broader basis than heretofore, so that greater economy will be exercised in use of funds and more cattle owners will benefit by the state and federal appropriations to combat this disease, according to plans of the state veterinarian. While tuberculosis eradication will continue as heretofore and a single breeder can have his herd tested, the work will be reduced to a minimum; and instead the area work will be pushed, whereby a whole community, such as a township, can be accredited and finally a county, and we trust the entire state.
>
> Area testing is not new. Adjoining states, such as Pennsylvania and Michigan, have been cleaning up their territory on this plan; Tennessee is also following such a program; and even Idaho finds it practicable in the range country. The report published in The Ohio Farmer last week of the clean-up just across the state line in Pennsylvania illustrates what will be followed in Ohio.
>
> **Ohio Has 1,000 Accredited Herds.**
>
> To date there are more than 1,000 accredited herds here in Ohio and when funds were available to feel safe and ought to be willing to employ their own veterinarian and bear the expense themselves from now on, after the state has set them squarely on their feet. So they have sent out to owners of accredited herds a letter stating it will hereafter be the policy of the state to eradicate bovine tuberculosis as rapidly and economically as possible and to extend the service to those who have heretofore been unable to have their herds tested.
>
> **The New Policy.**
>
> They are therefore asking that such accredited tuberculosis-free herds be tested annually hereafter by an accredited veterinarian (one approved by the state) at the owner's expense, such test to be made strictly in accordance with instructions heretofore followed in accredited herd plan testing. The state furnishes the tuberculin. No indemnity is given for reactors in such cases.
>
> About 100 accredited herds have been authorized to be tested by local veterinarians under this ruling. Once-tested herds will be taken care of after July 1, but any tests made up to that date will be only on condition of a waiver for indemnity.
>
> thus has a large majority of the breeders signed up to test their herds, the state will send there two veterinarians and they can quickly cover the whole area and pick out the reactors. The testing, the indemnity, the slaughter of reactors under federal inspection, all will be the same as formerly done for the individual. The only essential difference will be in accrediting groups or communities where heretofore the governmental authorities dealt only with the individual.
>
> Such a plan will go into operation this coming July. The plans are now being laid and organizations are already being perfected in several counties to carry out this program. This information and agreements have been distributed to many counties which have shown keen interest and immediate willingness to co-operate in such area testing.
>
> **No Indemnity For Scrub Bulls.**
>
> Indemnity will be paid on a scale similar to that heretofore in use by the state and federal departments. However, no indemnity will be paid for steers, sterile cows or grade bulls. A bull that reacts to the tuberculin test must have a registration certificate or no indemnity will be paid. What good is he anyhow, except for bologna and why should the state pay anything

The Ohio Farmer, *June 2, 1923 (Ohio Historical Society)*

and inefficient livestock sanitary laws as they relate to dairy inspection as Ohio. That as a result of said lax sanitary dairy inspection laws, Ohio has become a public mart where tubercular dairy cattle are bought and sold with perfect safety and their milk product likewise . . .

Three years later, OVMA President Dr. Reuben Hilty lamented the "very, very slow progress" in the control of bovine tuberculosis and also castigated towns and cities for their failure to take precautions:

> Why a municipality should, in the light of present-day knowledge on these all-important subjects, still allow the sale of raw milk from tuberculous cows is more than I can understand.

In his remarks, Dr. Hilty also said that "the world still awaits a genius who will evolve a plan . . . which will afford some hope of final victory." The same year, 1917, a plan was evolved. The United States Bureau of Animal Industry established its Tuberculosis Eradication Division and launched a cooperative eradication program based on the accredited herd plan, an accredited herd being one in which no tuberculosis was found in two annual or three semi-annual tests. It was what concerned veterinarians and others had been waiting for; within two years, the new plan was operating in 45 states, including Ohio. The battle against bovine tuberculosis had been joined in earnest.

But there was no overnight triumph; victory was years away. There were millions of head of livestock to be tested, opposition to the slaughtering of infected animals, and frequently a shortage of money. The latter was particularly troublesome in Ohio, as OVMA President Dr. Claude H. Case noted in his 1922 Annual Meeting remarks:

> We cannot make progress if, during the year, we test only 5 percent of the cattle scattered all over one state. To accomplish this, we must have appropriations and when we compare the paltry $50,000 given by our great state to the $350,000 given by the state of Iowa, is it any wonder that we cannot test any new herd in Ohio, when the owners are clamoring for tests of their herds . . . I say it is a shame for Ohio to retard this great work; every veterinarian in Ohio should make it a point to see his representative, have his clients see him, and demand that Ohio appropriate the money it should . . .

The membership responded and throughout this crucial period the OVMA played a critical role in

> ## THE OHIO FARMER
>
> # First Counties Are Tuberculosis Free
>
> ### Four Entire Ohio Communities Rid Cattle Of Dread Disease
>
> #### By L. L. RUMMELL
>
> [Erie], Huron and Medina counties are the first communities in Ohio to finish their campaigns on the area plan for eradication of tuberculosis among cattle. Starting [in 19]14 the federal department of agriculture [sent] additional veterinarians into four Ohio [coun]ties: Erie, Huron, Medina and Allen; the [plan] being to demonstrate an extensive drive in [tuber]culin testing by having a veterinarian in [each] township.
>
> [Vete]rinarians assigned to Wayne, Fulton and [other] counties were temporarily withdrawn to [aid] in these four counties. These counties [were] selected for an intensive eradication cam[paign] because road conditions were relatively [favor]able for the work, the counties were fairly [well] organized, and the herd owners were ready [to off]er the co-operation necessary.
>
> [All]en County would also have finished had [not t]hree federal veterinarians been withdrawn [and sent] to California to help in the campaign [waged] against foot and mouth disease.
>
> ["The] spirit of co-operation in these counties [was] wonderful," declared Dr. F. A. Zimmer, [state] veterinarian, "and we had very few ob[jector]s, and they were largely folks who were [not] veterinarians. This is the prime essential to proper conduct of the work, for this preliminary educational work must be done by the local agencies and not by the veterinarians themselves. The keynote to the situation in every county is this close co-operation with the herd owner and his willingness to accept the indemnity provision for reactors.
>
> That this area plan rightly conducted is fruitful of results in eradicating this diseases among herds of cattle is well brought out by the experience of Lyme Township, Huron County. There about a year ago the farmers organized themselves to rid their herds of the disease, and they made their first tests, followed by good sanitary measures in cases where tuberculosis was found. Reactors were taken out of the herds and the premises disinfected. This year when the state and federal veterinarians went over this same territory they found only one single tubercular animal, and this reactor was an animal that came in from the outside without a test.
>
> #### Protection From Outside Infestation
>
> Such a case also bears evidence to the fact that once a territory is put on the modified [...] tested are placed under quarantine, and in some localities they are not able now to sell their milk or cattle.
>
> Looking ahead into the future of this work and its possibilities for 1925, Dr. Zimmer says that four essentials are paramount:
>
> (1) We need proper laws here in Ohio to supplant some of the now obsolete statutes regarding this work. Some states have a provision by law whereby the county commissioners in any county can pay the expenses incident to testing, if 60 percent of the herd owners sign up; and then when 75 percent sign up, the others can be forced to test whether they want to or not. Iowa, Wisconsin, Michigan, Illinois and other states have such provisions.
>
> (2) The close co-operation of herd owners local agencies, state veterinarian's office and federal department is necessary.
>
> (3) More veterinarians to handle the work Today we have only 12 state veterinarians, some of them on part time, and eight federal inspectors. This is hardly sufficient for the present work, and there are 27 counties, some well organized, others partly organized, waiting pa tiently and otherwise for their turn to come.
>
> (4) More adequate appropriations.

The Ohio Farmer, *May 24, 1924 (Ohio Historical Society)*

pressing for adequate funding of the state's tuberculosis eradication program. In 1924, State Veterinarian Dr. Fred Zimmer could report:

> ... the plan has enlarged until at present there are almost 1,200 accredited herds in Ohio with approximately 3,900 herds under supervision scattered in various counties that have had one or more tests.

The following year Zimmer, who was the recognized leader of the eradication effort, scored a victory that assured continued progress. He secured passage of legislation fully confirming the state's authority to carry out the program. Until then there had been some serious legal questions which tended to strengthen the opposition. Commenting on the new law in 1926, the OVMA Legislative Committee observed:

> Ohio has one of the best laws in the United States upon which will be built the foundation for the complete eradication of tuberculosis from our herds of cattle.

A sizable number of veterinarians were directly involved in the eradication program. In 1925, there were 25 veterinarians working full-time and another 14 involved four days a week on a per diem basis. In addition, five counties also were employing veterinarians to test herds.

But, obviously this was not enough; the scope of the effort required the involvement of the entire profession. State Veterinarian Zimmer, addressing the OVMA in 1926, told members that:

> The veterinary practitioner stands in an important relation to the organization in carrying out the eradication plan and as the work progresses ... he will be asked to assume increased responsibilities. In all probability, state and federal appropriations will never be sufficient to obtain enough regularly employed veterinarians to more than blaze the trail in eradicating TB....

Again, Ohio's veterinarians responded and private practitioners assumed a major role in eradication efforts. Through their involvement, they also were instrumental in blunting opposition and gaining increased public acceptance of the program.

Early on, resistance in some quarters had been strong. Although farmers were compensated for slaughtered cattle, many resisted the destruction of their herds; in some instances veterinarians arriving to test animals were escorted off the premises at gunpoint and, on at least one occasion, a veterinary proponent of eradication was bodily ejected from a farm meeting. But as the program evolved, attitudes changed and much of the credit for this must go to the educational efforts of OVMA members and other veterinarians. In 1929, the Association's Progress and Education committee reported that "thrifty and progressive cattle owners" had a positive attitude toward the eradication program and that despite some continued opposition, "steady progress" was being made.

This program continued for the next three years and in 1932 a milestone was reached. It was announced at the OVMA Annual Meeting that:

> ... in December it was recommended that Ohio be placed on the list of the modified accredited states. In this list Ohio occupies fifth place and Wisconsin will be next on the list, which is made up as follows: North Carolina, first; Maine, second; Michigan, third; Indiana, fourth.... Every herd of cattle in the state has been tested and so far as is known, no county in the state has over .5 percent infection. This is a project in which every veterinarian in the state has played a part and one in which we should all take a great deal of pride.

The battle against bovine tuberculosis was being won. And over the same period in which it was fought, veterinary medicine also waged parallel campaigns against other costly and destructive animal diseases.

One target was hog cholera. While not a direct threat to human health and therefore less dramatic than bovine tuberculosis, hog cholera was nonetheless a costly burden for the American farmer. In the mid-teens of the 20th Century, the smoke from burning hogs rose from the roadsides of Ohio and the following years were marked by recurring outbreaks of the disease; Ohio had a major one in 1926 and an outbreak of even greater proportions in 1932. That year, the OVMA's Committee on Disease reported:

> There is still much to be learned about hog cholera, particularly in regards to the means by which it is spread.

Protective vaccination was the answer but it could be a double-edged sword. Handled by professionals it was effective, but when undertaken by laymen it was often a futile exercise. Indeed "lay" vaccination and the feeding of garbage to hogs were considered the principal causes of the disease. A major aim of the OVMA in the campaign against hog cholera was to discourage "lay" vaccination; the Association sought

The Ohio Farmer, *October 30, 1926* (Ohio Historical Society)

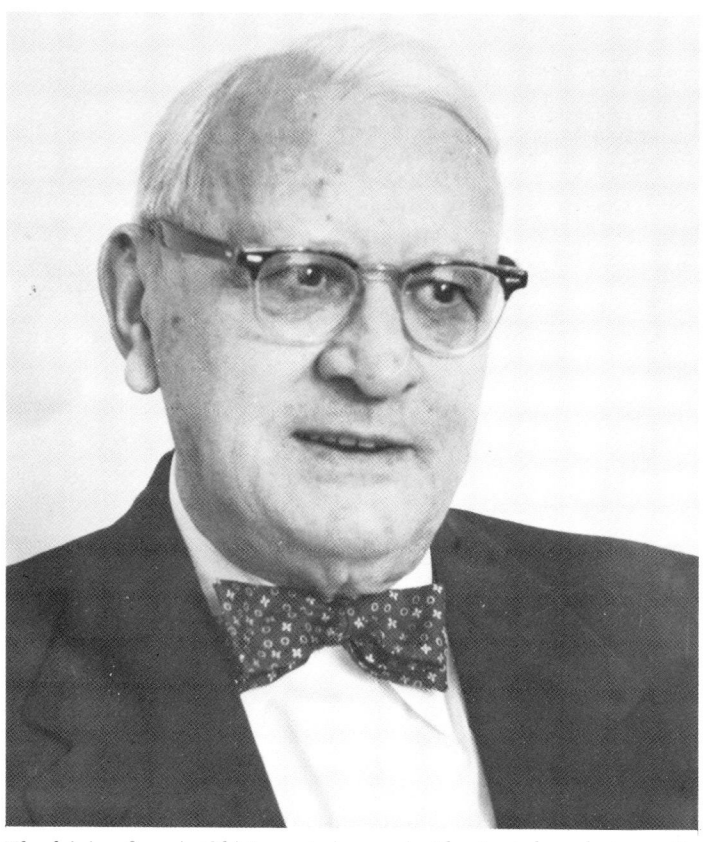

The driving force in Ohio's campaign against bovine tuberculosis was Dr. Fred Zimmer, another OVMA leader who served as State Veterinarian from 1923-29 and again from 1935-39. Zimmer was OVMA president in 1931. (OVMA files)

both legal rulings and legislative action to restrain the practice. In this effort to assure professional vaccination it won the support of *The Ohio Farmer*, which in an editorial of April 14, 1928, stated:

> This is the time of year farmers are thinking about vaccinating their spring pig crop, safeguarding it against any possible outbreak of cholera later in the season. Ohio went through the fire two years ago. We don't want to get burnt again through carelessness.... Consult your local veterinarian. You will usually find him a pretty helpful fellow.... Few indeed are the farmers qualified to handle serum and virus; *it is a job for the trained veterinarian.*

The editorial was further confirmation of the growing prestige of the professional veterinarian. "Lay" vaccination and garbage "dinners" were to continue to complicate efforts to stamp out hog cholera in the decades ahead, but eventually scientific veterinary care would prevail. As with bovine tuberculosis, hog cholera's years, if not its days, were numbered.

Another target for eradication was brucellosis; it was a threat to the health of humans as well as animals. A concerted effort to eliminate this disease began in the 1930s and OVMA President Dr. John Jackman commented on the campaign at the 1936 Annual Meeting:

> In the past year many new projects were de-

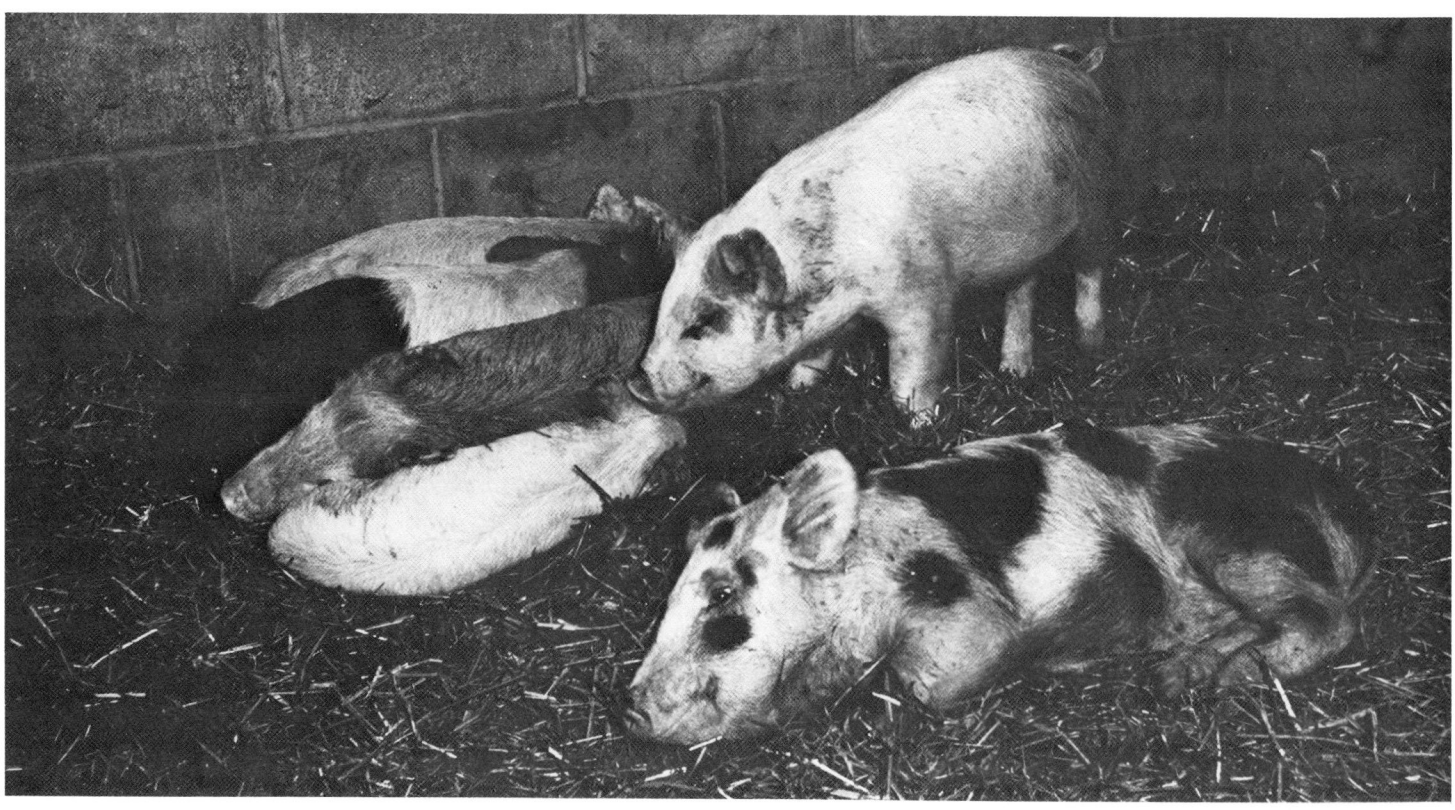

One of the most costly and destructive of livestock diseases was hog cholera. First identified in Ohio in 1833, it continued to plague farmers for nearly a century and a half. (Ohio Veterinary Medical Board)

veloped in which the veterinary profession played a part. I refer, principally, to the program of the federal government in its attempt to control and eliminate Bang's Disease. This project alone employed the majority of our recent graduates, as well as many others. We recognize that this program will entail the spending of more money and greater efforts than was required for the eradication of Tuberculosis.

(Jackman himself was painfully familiar with the disease; he contracted it while treating cows at a Columbus dairy. Milk from the dairy, incidentally, was sold to the county tuberculosis hospital.)

The brucellosis campaign, like other eradication programs, was a long-term effort; as late as the mid-1940s, 15 to 18 percent of Ohio herds were still infected and the disease cost farmers up to $150 million a year in calf and milk losses. But veterinary campaigners were persistent and they enlisted allies, including the Ohio Medical Association. The latter venture, reflective of the growing ties between human and animal medicine, was described in a 1949 report of the OVMA's Public Health Committee:

(Three veterinarians), Dr. Edgington, Dr. Geyer, and Dr. Greenlee were appointed to cooperate with the Ohio Medical Association and carry out plans for disseminating information relative to the veterinary aspects of brucellosis ... the

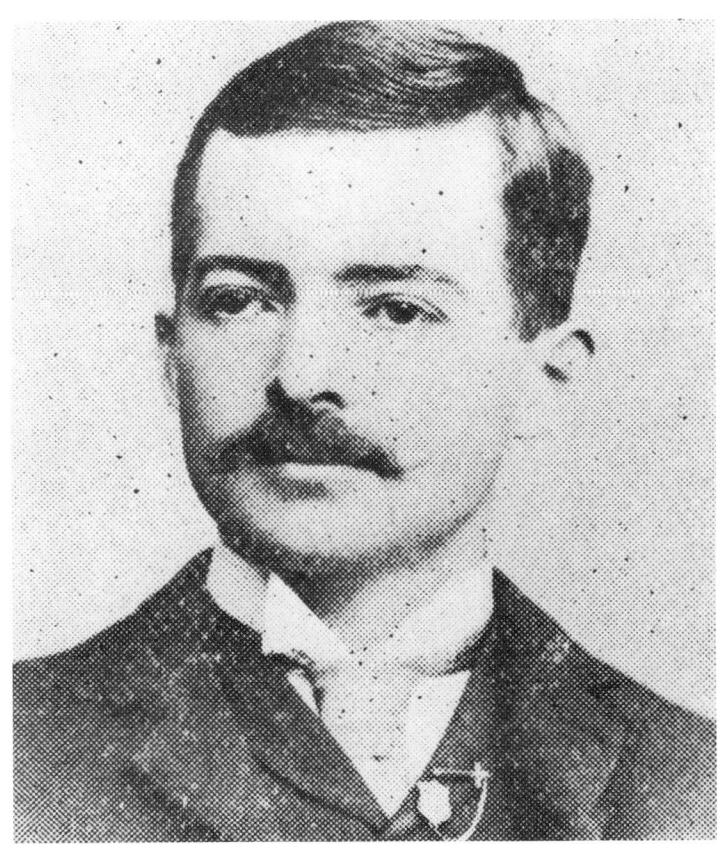

Dr. Mark Francis, the first graduate of the OSU College of Veterinary Medicine. Francis became Dean of the School of Veterinary Medicine at Texas A & M and played a major role in the campaign to eradicate Texas fever. (Photo Archives, Ohio State University)

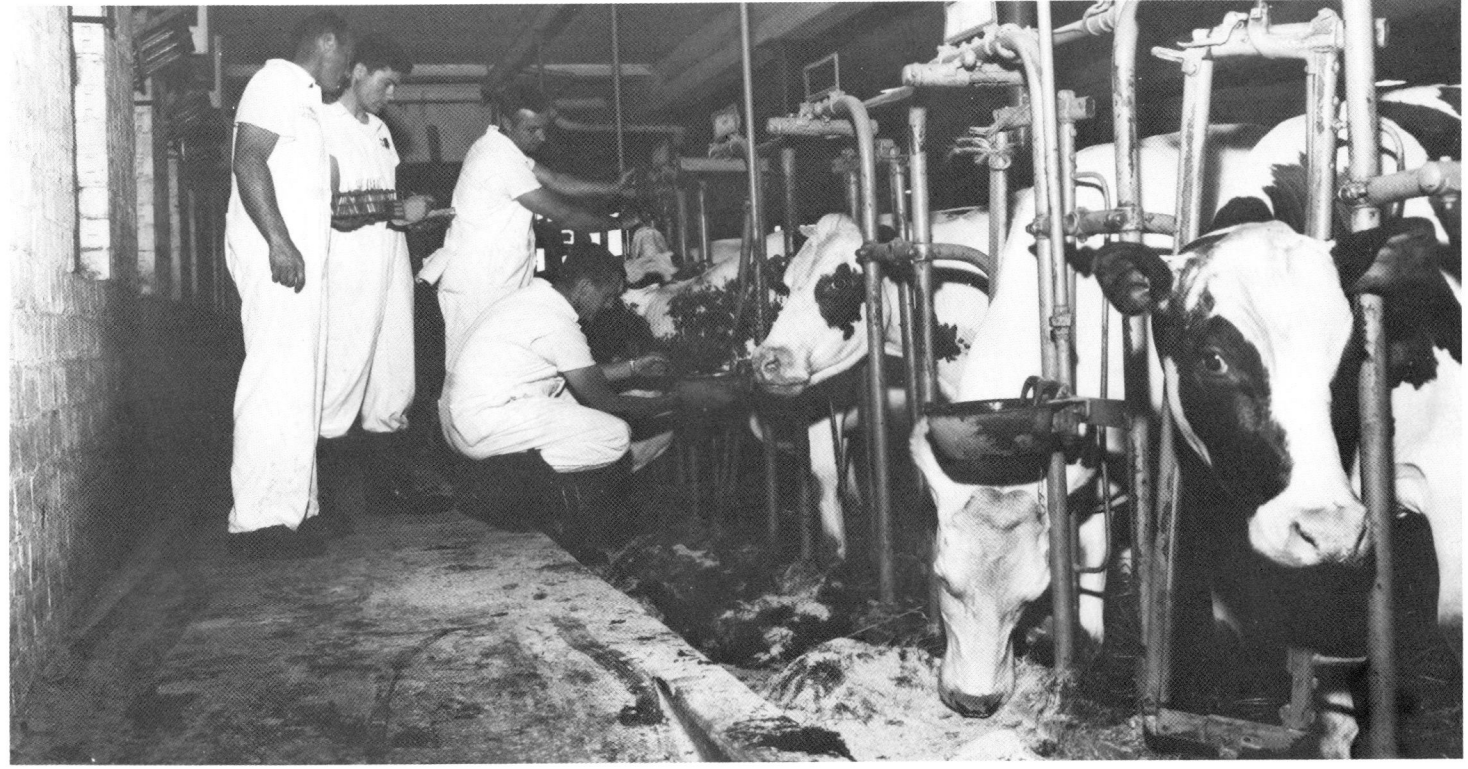

Comprehensive testing programs like this scene from 1960 were the key to the eradication of bovine diseases by the mid-1970s in Ohio. (Photo Archives, Ohio State University)

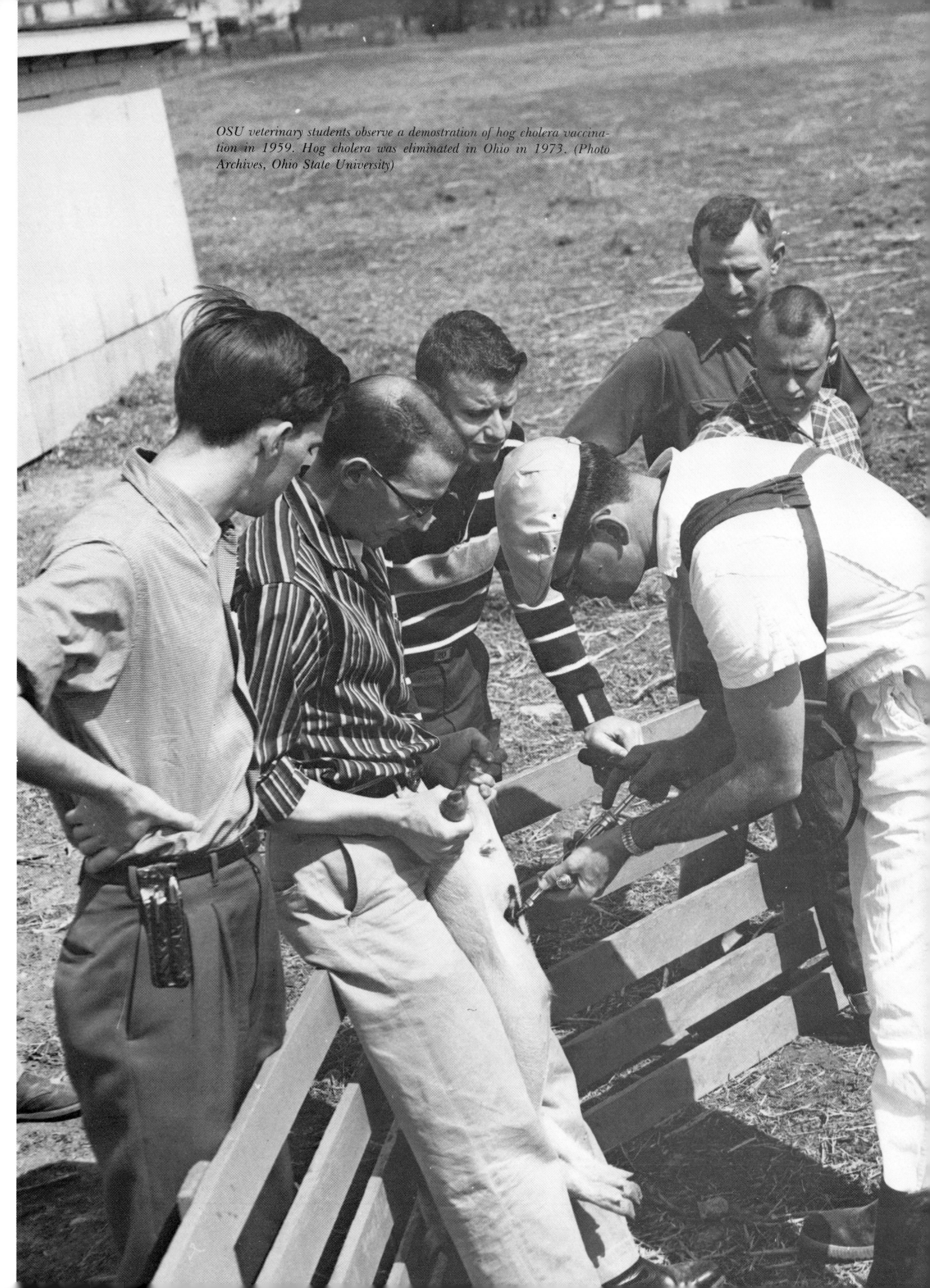

OSU veterinary students observe a demostration of hog cholera vaccination in 1959. Hog cholera was eliminated in Ohio in 1973. (Photo Archives, Ohio State University)

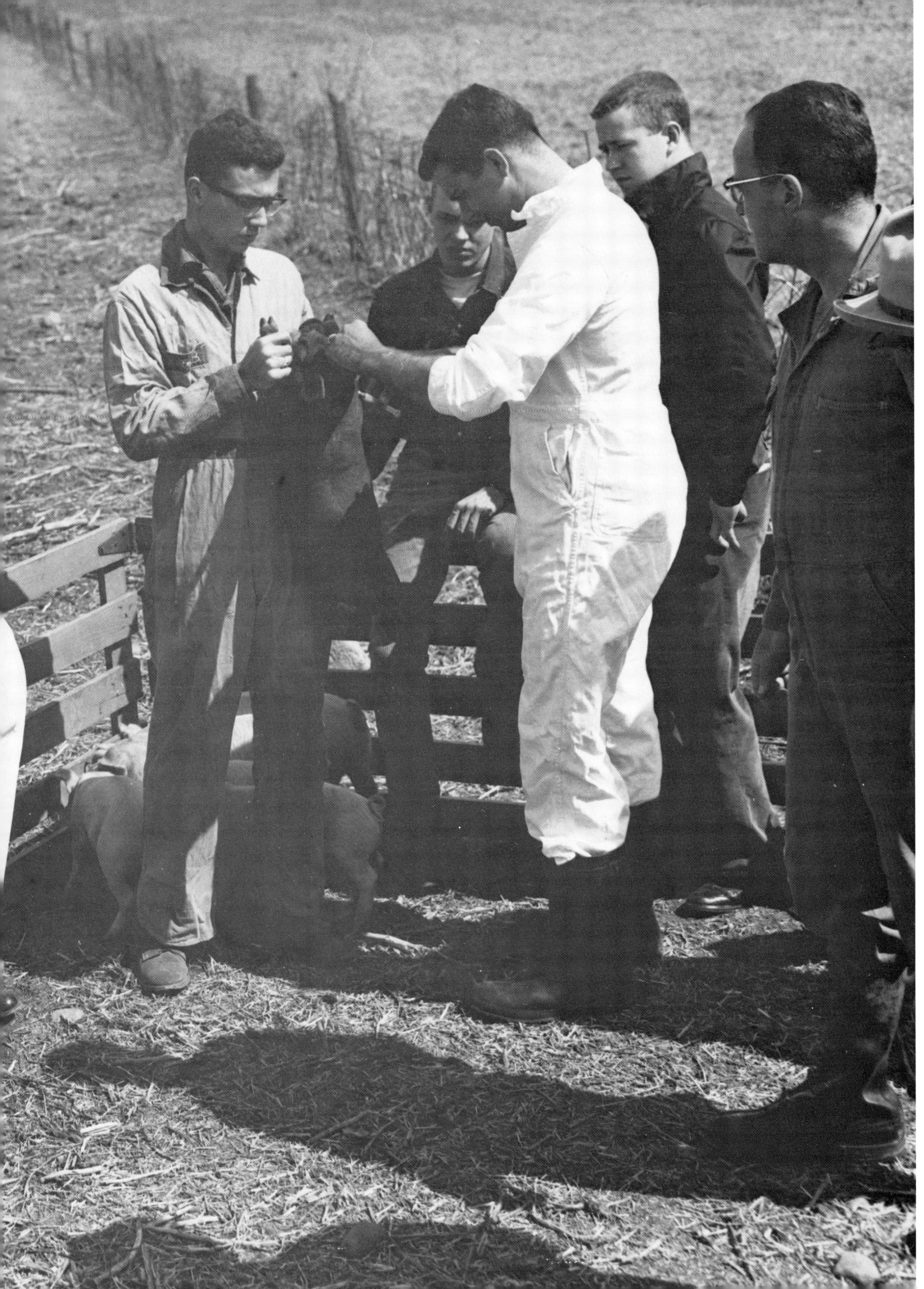

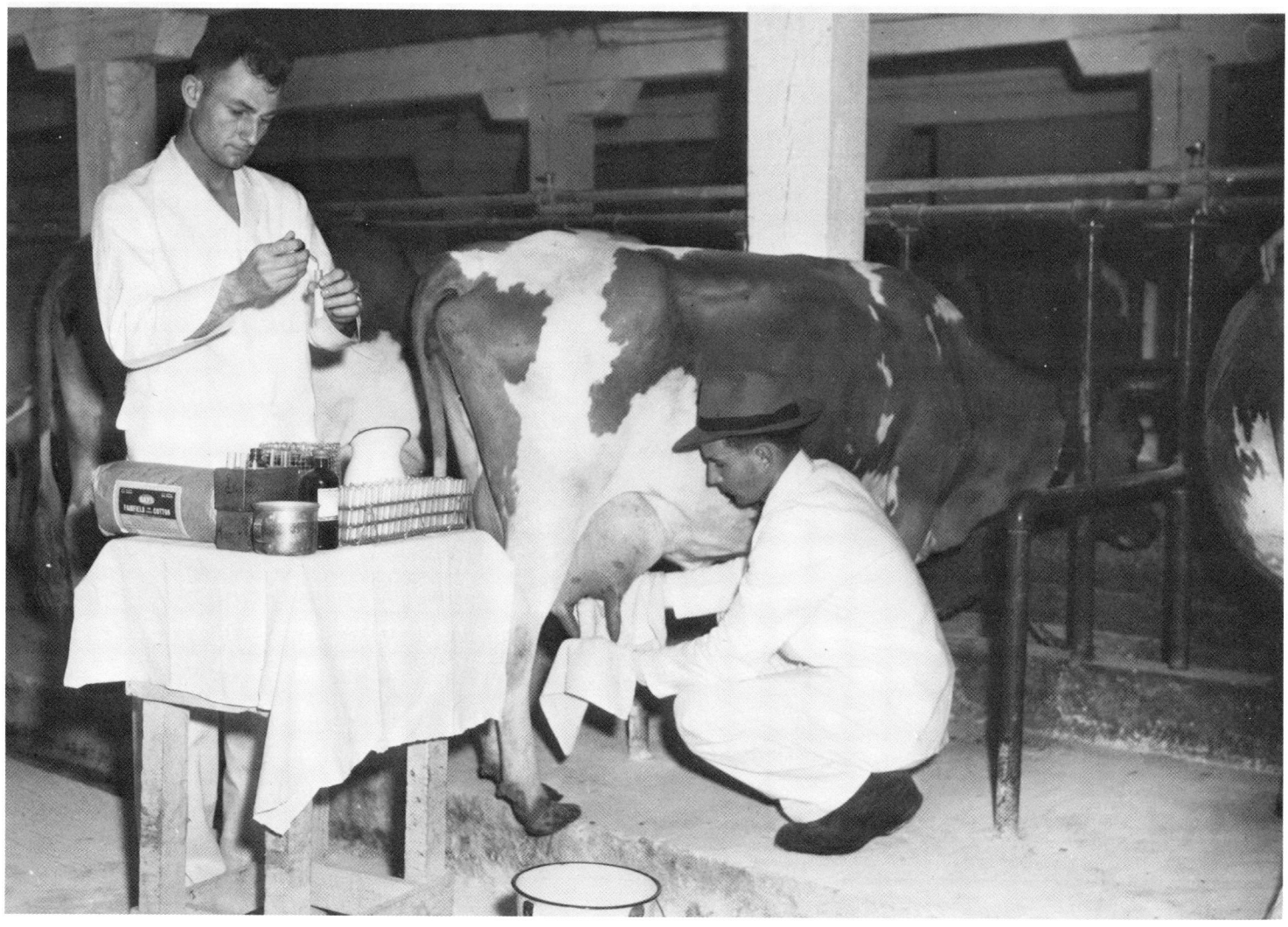

Scenes from the 1960s: OSU veterinary students testing cattle for tuberculosis, brucellosis and other diseases. Continued testing prevents a recurrence of the devastating plagues of the past. (Photo Archives, Ohio State University)

brucellosis publicity program carried out jointly by the Ohio Medical Association and the Ohio State Veterinary Medical Association has been very effective. It has not only stimulated interest in the public health aspects of the disease but has increased demand for brucellosis control programs among livestock.

Overall, Ohio veterinarians spent more than a half century battling bovine tuberculosis, hog cholera and brucellosis. The efforts were costly, time-consuming, and on many occasions, frustrating. But in time the diseases yielded to veterinary science: in 1948 Ohio was officially designed as an accredited tuberculosis-free state, in 1972 it was declared brucellosis-free, and in 1973 hog cholera was eliminated. Equally successful efforts have resulted in the control and/or eradication of other afflictions, including foot-and-mouth disease, anthrax and scabies, to cite only a few. There are still isolated recurrences of some diseases, but these can be quickly controlled and the devastating plagues of earlier years are no more.

A step back into the past is necessary at this point to round out this brief history of disease control efforts. No report would be complete without note of the contributions of Dr. Mark Francis to the eradication of Texas cattle fever. A prize student of Dr. H.J. Detmers and the first graduate of the OSU College of Veterinary Medicine, Francis spent most of his career in Texas, where he became Dean of the School of Veterinary Medicine at Texas A & M. Although for years his work was overshadowed by the achievements of Dr. D.E. Salmon, chief of the U.S. Bureau of Animal Industry, he is now recognized as a pioneer in the fight against Texas fever and is credited by Smithcors with being "largely responsible for the improvement of the Texas cattle industry." One measure of his stature is the tribute paid him by OSU President W.O. Thompson, who was quoted in a 1924 issue of the *Ohio State University Monthly* as remarking that, "If Ohio State had done nothing else except give Dr. Francis to the world, her mission has been worthwhile."

Hundreds of Ohio veterinarians, both honored and unsung, deserve similar tribute. So does the OVMA as an organization. The writers of the 1970 Association history put it best when they said:

> The success of all these (disease eradication) programs would never have been possible without an enlightened, alert profession who constitute the first line of defense . . . when disease problems gain entrance into our livestock population. Without our OVMA, which provided the main source of continuing education for many years and the opportunity for group dialogue to iron out our differences of opinion, animal health in Ohio and throughout the rest of the United States would not be on the high plane it is today.

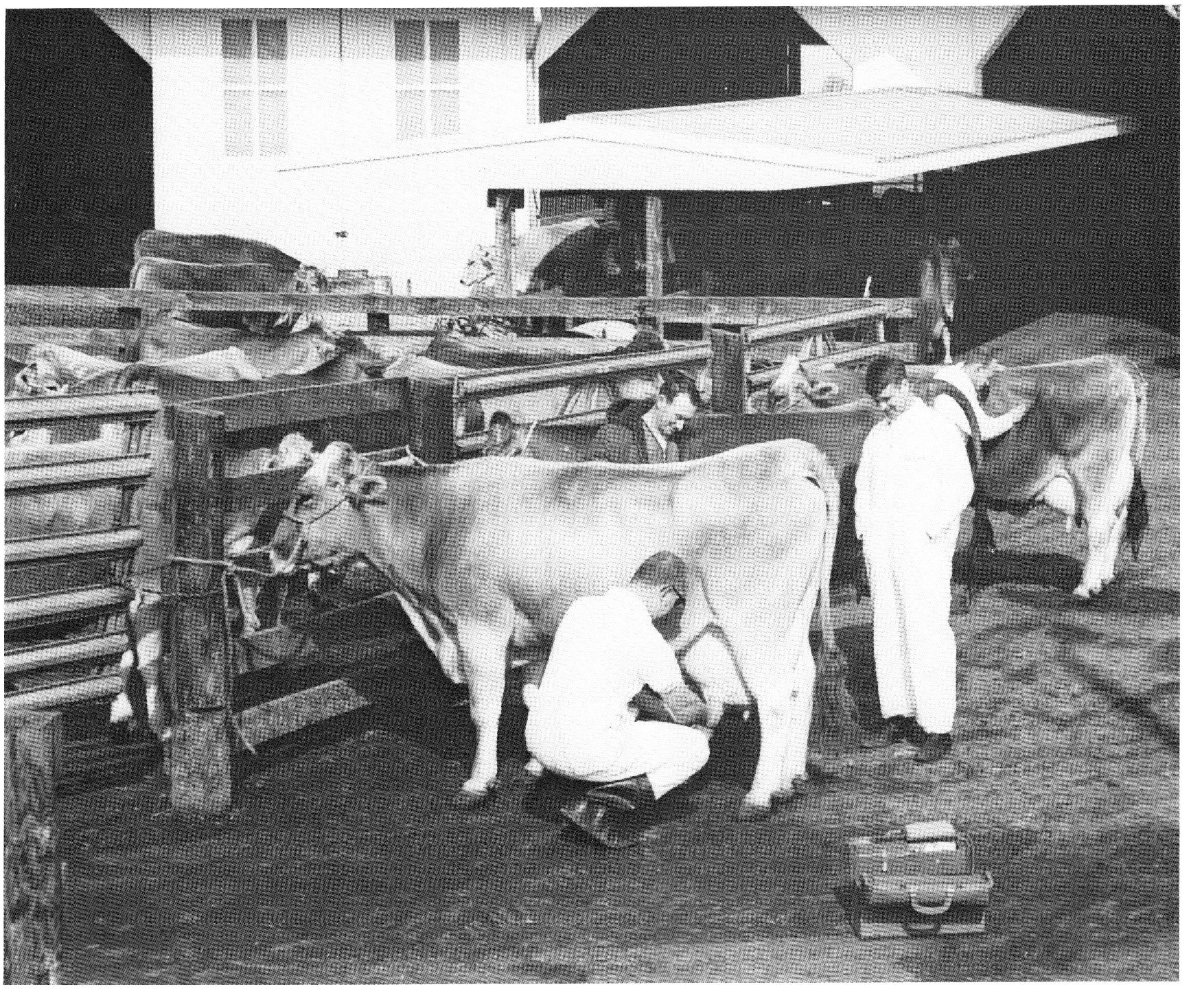

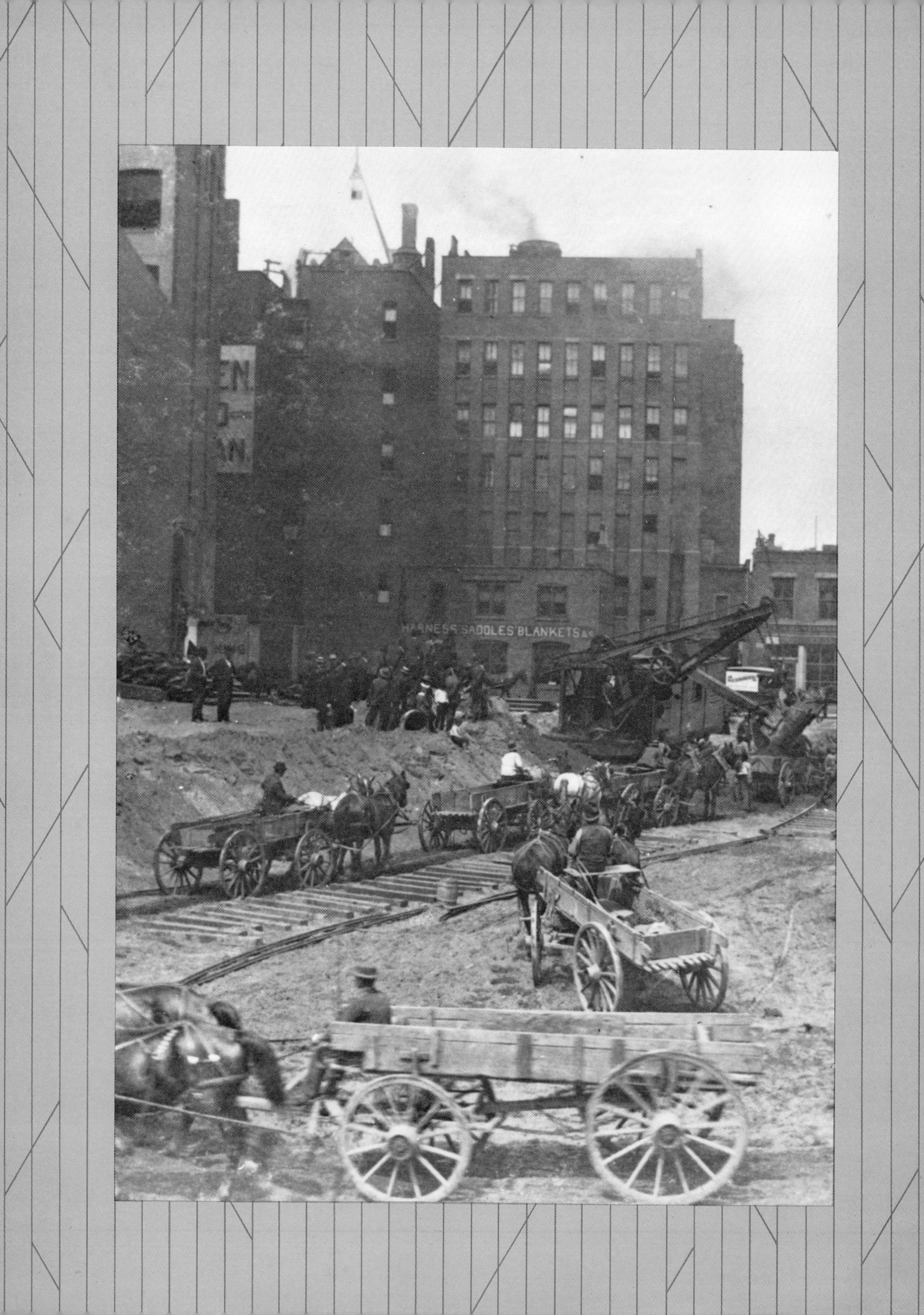

CHAPTER V

THE 20s AND 30s;
NEW CONCERNS & OPPORTUNITIES

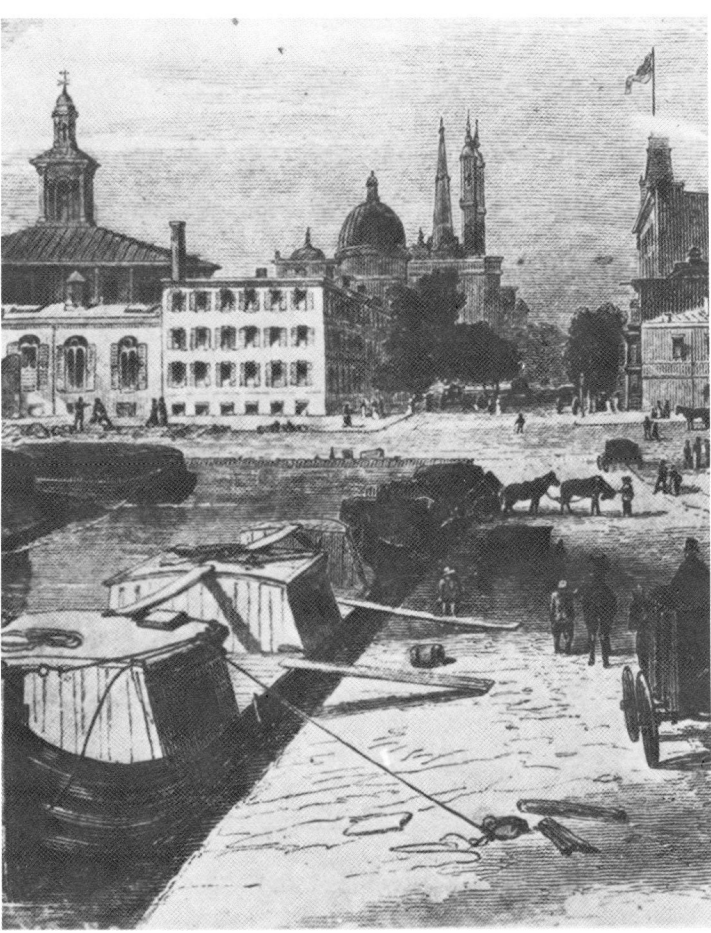

The horse was an urban as well as rural king. Even water transportation via canal boat depended on horse power, as this 1860 Cincinnati scene illustrates. It would be another 60 years before the reign of the urban workhorse came to an end. (Ohio Historical Society)

Workhorses at a construction site in Cleveland, 1898. (Cleveland Public Library)

The campaigns against the great epizootic diseases which highlighted the 1920s and succeeding decades greatly enhanced the stature of the professional veterinarian. In the same period other events also had a strong impact on the profession, altering the course of veterinary education and the careers of many practitioners.

The first of these events was anticipated in a casual remark made by the Mayor of Columbus in 1914. Welcoming members at the OVMA's 30th Annual Meeting, George J. Karb said:

> I cannot tell you much about a horse. I used to be the owner of several very good horses, but since we have the automobile, I, like some other fellows, disposed of my horse.

In 1914, the handwriting was already on the wall. The day of the workhorse was drawing to a close, its termination signalled by the noisy rattle of the internal combustion engine and the cars and trucks it powered.

Initially, it was a slow process; the horse (and many of its human advocates) resisted the clattery advance of motorized vehicles. But by the 1920s the termination process was accelerating. An Akron veterinarian recalls that when he began practice in 1923, there were about 2,000 horses in the city hauling milk, coal, beer and dozens of other commodities. But then the horse began to disappear, very rapidly. "In three or four years, they just seemed to fade. The automobile just took charge."

This decline was also noted in 1924 by Dr. C. H. Stange, President of the AVMA. Addressing the OVMA Annual Meeting, he observed that:

> (In the past) veterinary practice was composed chiefly of horse practice. Ten to twelve years ago, 75 to 80 percent of the cases coming into clinics were horses; today (they comprise) less than 25 percent.... The horse today has largely ceased to be a means of transportation...

The abrupt fall of the horse from favor posed a serious challenge to the veterinary profession which had long placed heavy emphasis on equine practice. Alone, it had the makings of a calamity. But the demise of the workhorse was only one problem; in the same period the profession was confronted by a major agricultural depression and, only a few years later, by the national economic collapse which began with Black Thursday, 1929. Combined, these events generated powerful winds of change.

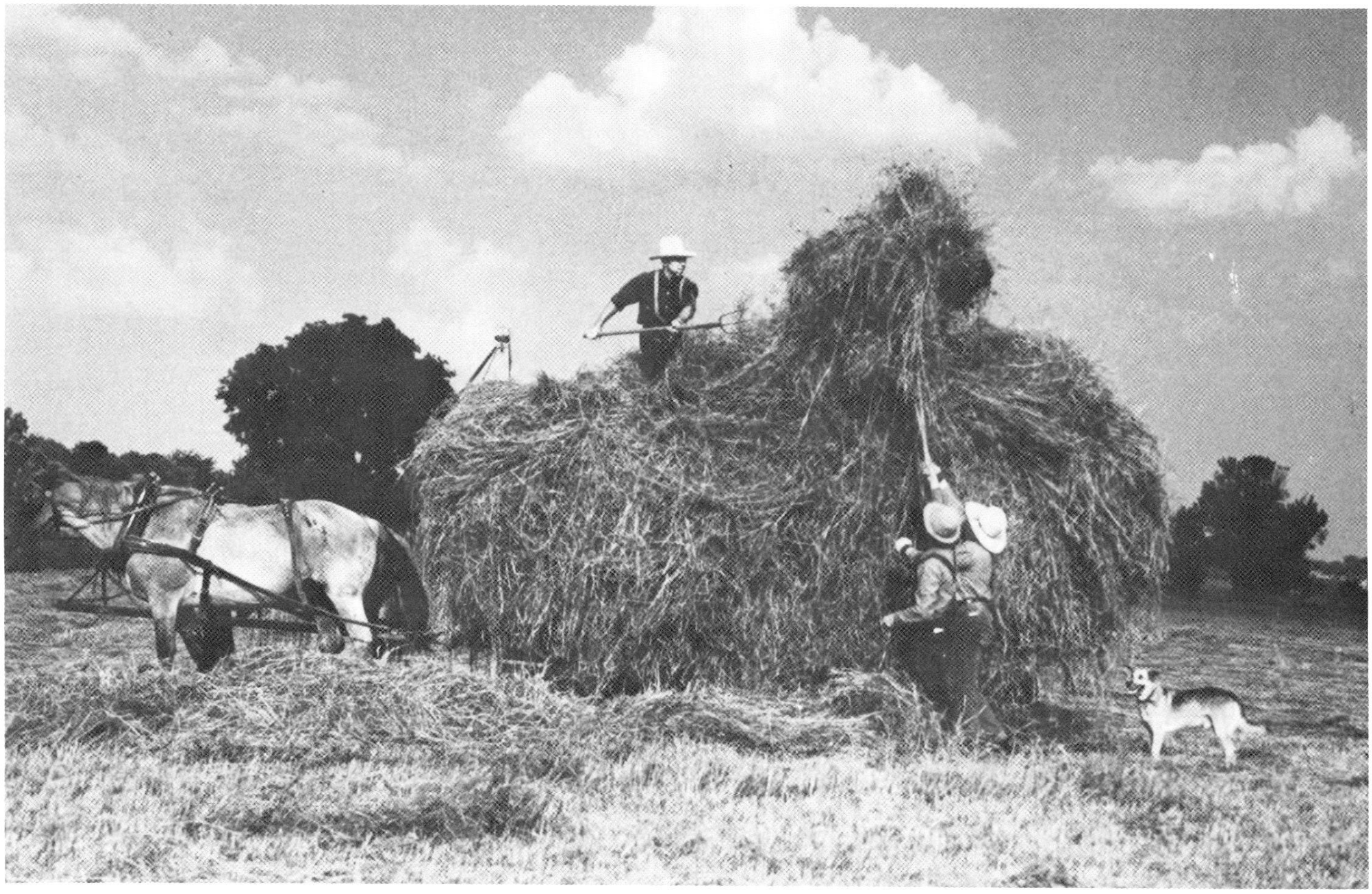

On farms, horse power remained a major energy source for years after the decline of the urban workhorse. In the mid and late 1930s, scenes like this still were common. (Top photo: Ohio Historical Society; bottom photo: Herbert Rebman)

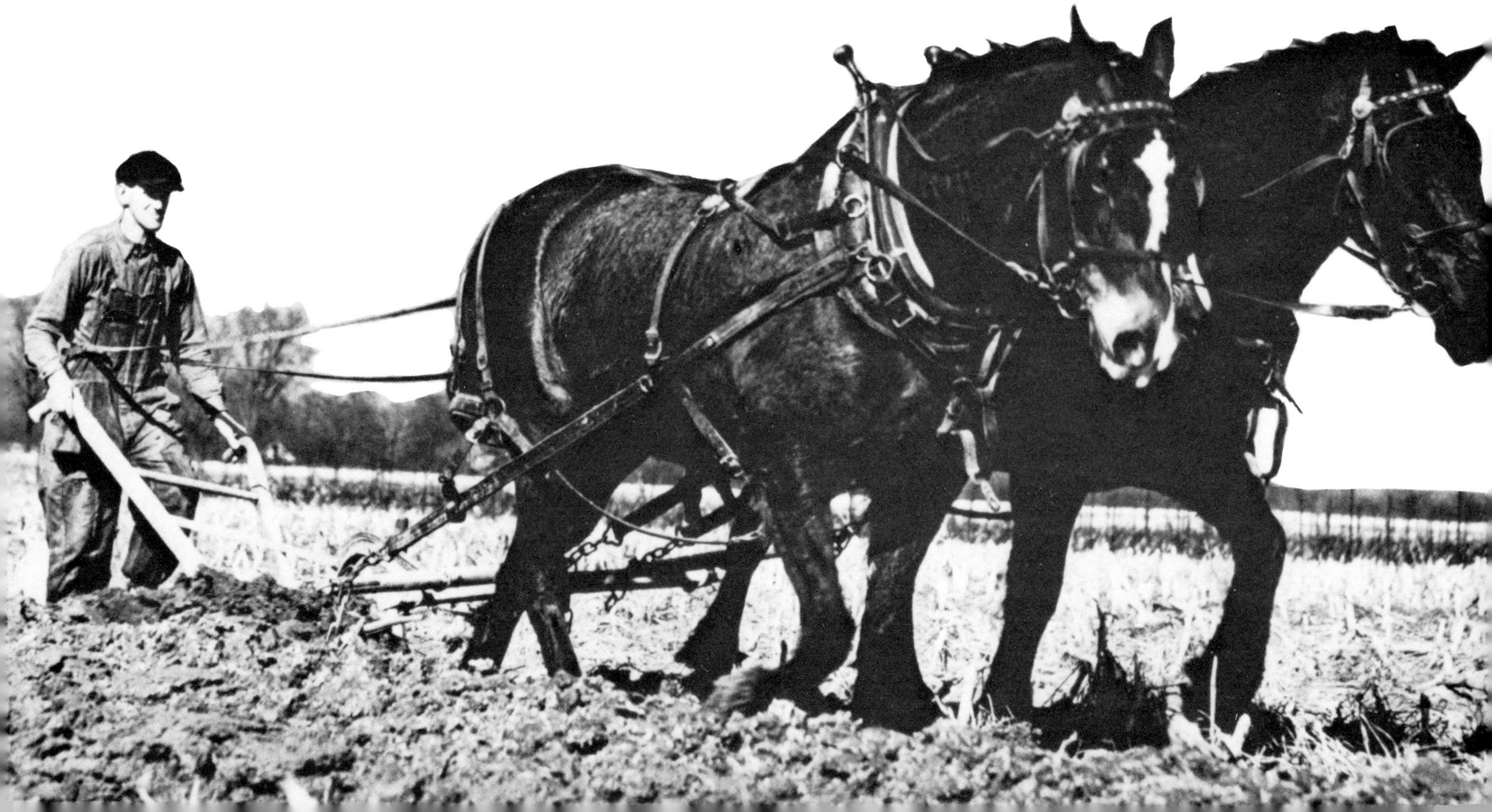

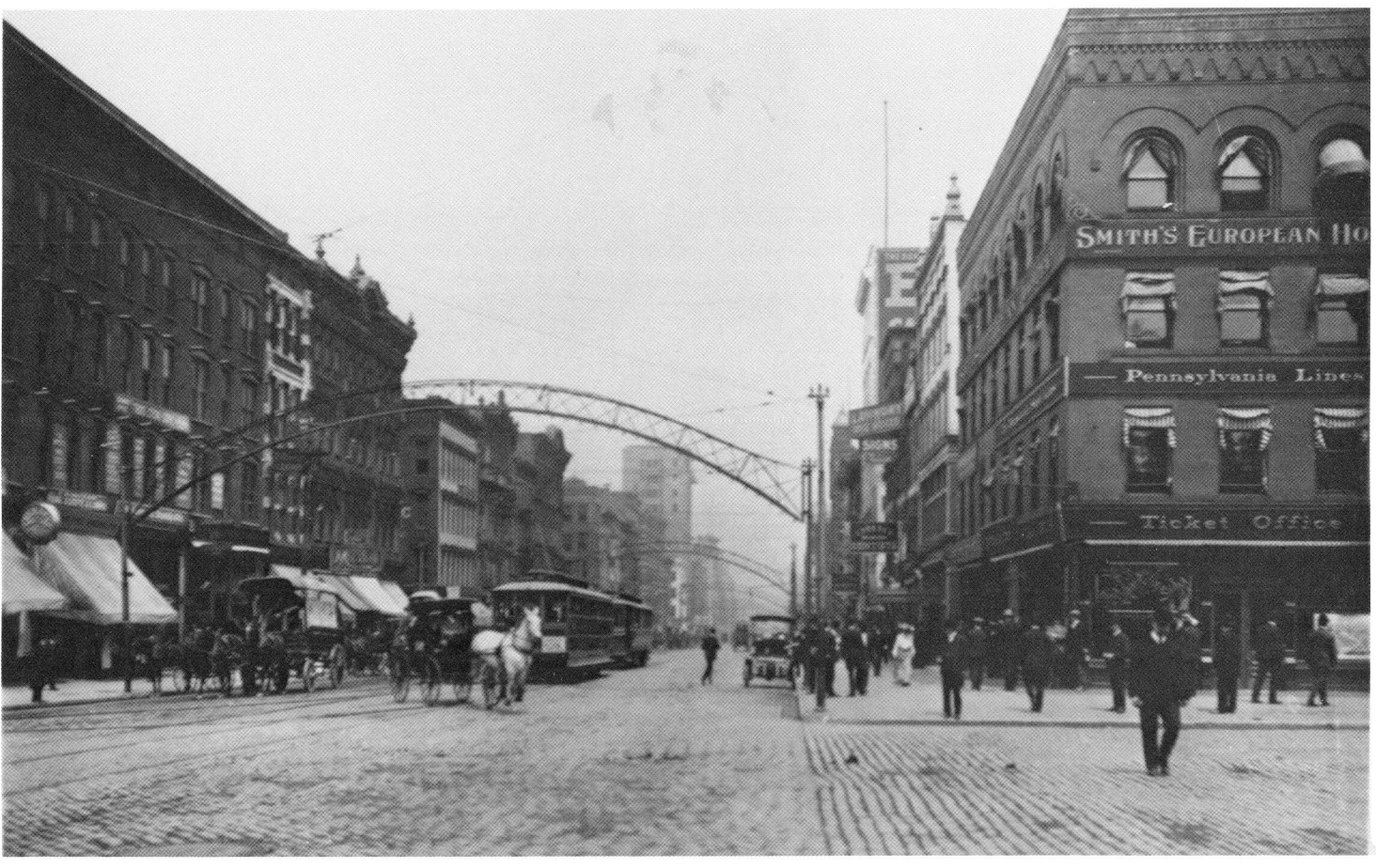

Columbus near the turn of the century. The streetcars were electric-powered now, but horse power still was essential for the movement of goods and people. (Library of Congress)

There were bound to be casualties and the first were the private veterinary schools. Already hard-pressed by competition from state-supported veterinary colleges, the private institutions were badly damaged by the shift from horse to motor power, since most of them were geared to meeting the urban needs for equine practitioners. Suddenly denied these markets, it became only a matter of time before they faded from the scene and the time allotted was a handful of years.

The final blow came in 1920 when the AVMA and the U.S. Bureau of Animal Industry mandated uniform requirements for entrance into veterinary schools and uniformity in the length and number of academic years for graduation. All schools had to meet these requirements, as well as new standards for facilities, faculty and courses of study, in order to be accredited.

The already-embattled private schools, totally dependent on student fees, now had to choose between drastically increasing fees and losing students or closing their doors. One by one they chose the latter. Ohio's only remaining private institution, the Cincinnati Veterinary College, went out of business in 1920 and seven years later the nation's last private school closed down. An era had ended.

The decline and fall of the private colleges was inevitable, given the changing scene. But in their time they made important contributions. Commenting on their passing, Dr. Arthur Schalk has written:

> Thus, after more than sixty years of valuable service to the nation's animal industry, a most timely and useful phase of American veterinary medical education came to a close.... Private schools performed a yeoman service. Our farm animals were increasing by millions yearly, and there would have been a definite scarcity of veterinary practitioners had not these private schools turned out large numbers of graduates.

The combination of events which sounded a death-knell for private institutions also impacted heavily on state-supported veterinary colleges; in fact, there were some who claimed to hear the same bells tolling for them. With the decline of horse power (and horse practice) and the serious agricultural depression, veterinary medicine did not seem to be a very promis-

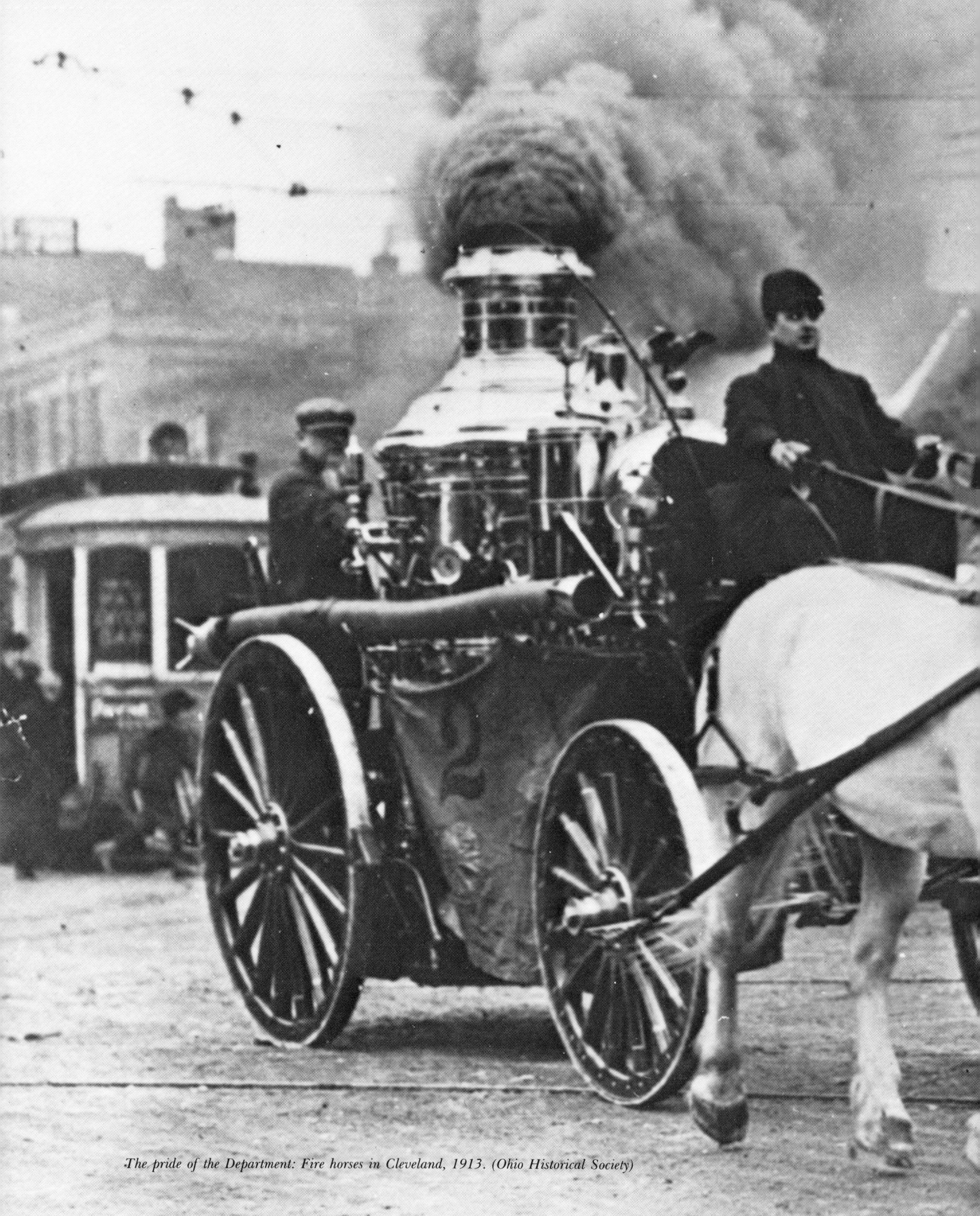
The pride of the Department: Fire horses in Cleveland, 1913. (Ohio Historical Society)

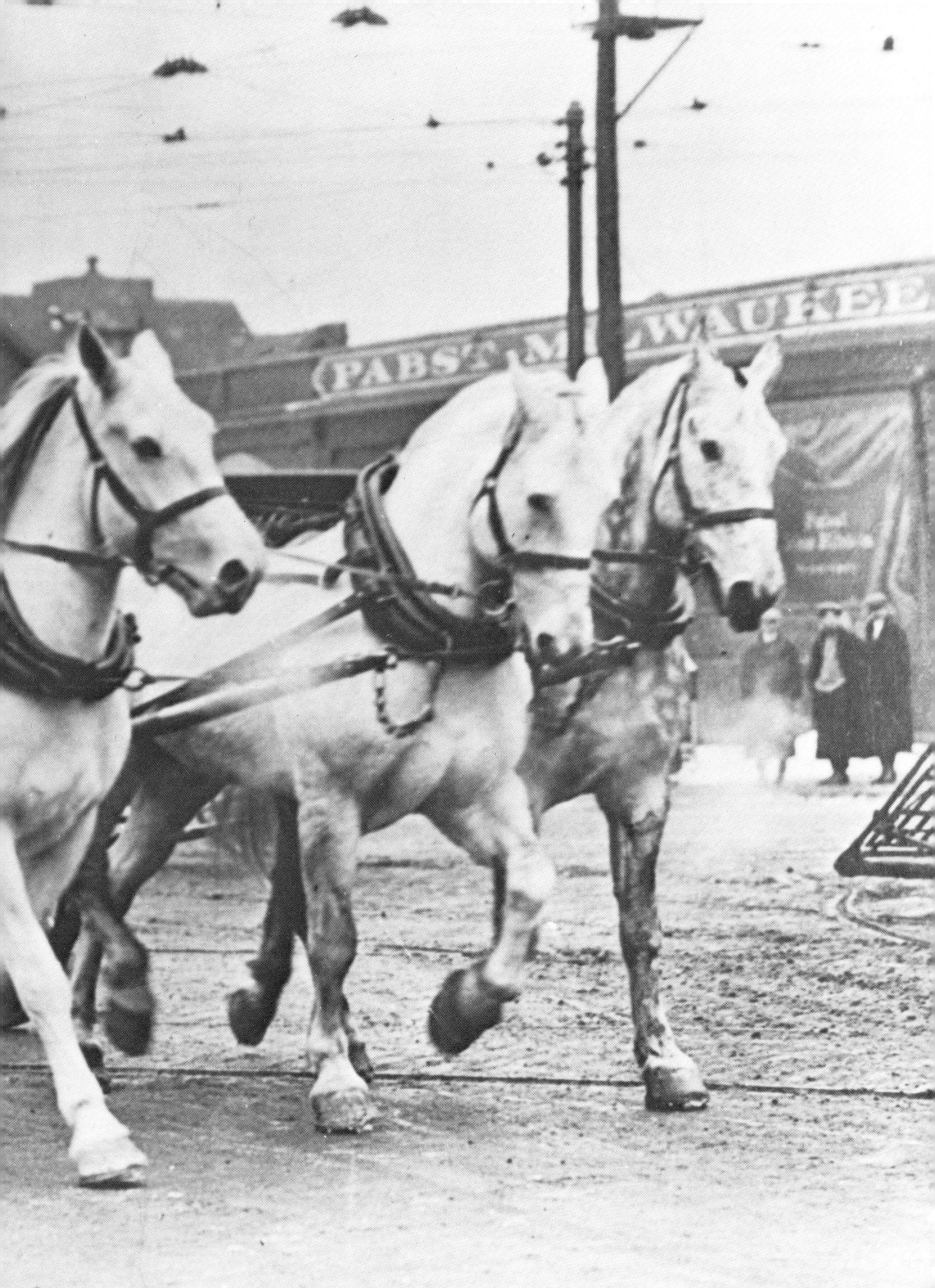

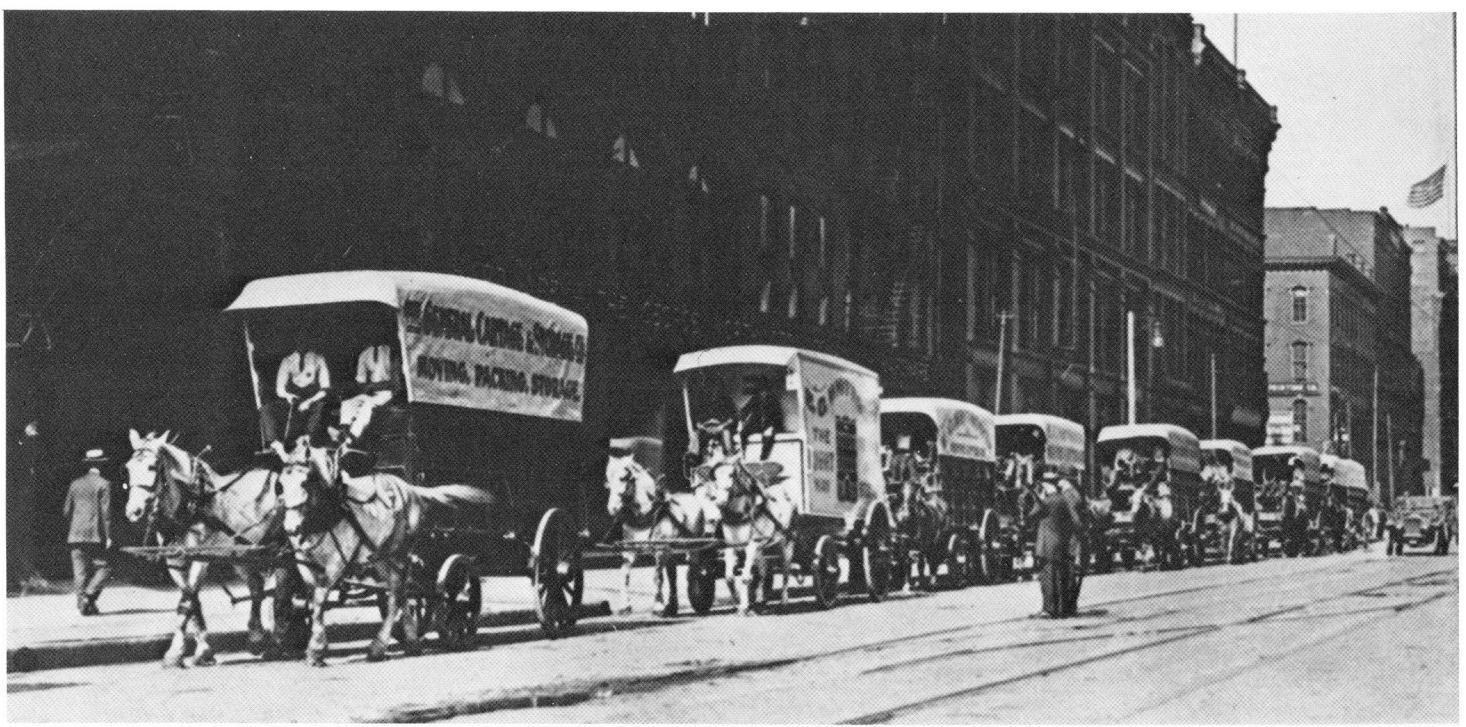

Cartage wagons on a Cleveland street. And coming up on the right, a noisy rival that would eventually triumph. (Ohio Historical Society)

ing profession. Student enrollments declined, sharply in many cases, and some colleges actually considered closing their doors. In 1921 the OVMA's Committee on Progress and Education warned the Annual Meeting that "the number of students in the veterinary colleges of America has declined to an alarming extent," noting that the OSU College of Veterinary Medicine had a total enrollment of 106, with only 18 in the freshman class.

Four years later, in 1925, the same committee's report was equally gloomy and apprehensive:

> There has been a decrease in the enrollment in veterinary schools during the past few years. The discouraging situation in agriculture may be responsible for this condition. At present there are 141 senior students enrolled in all the veterinary colleges of America. In 1916, there were about 3,000 students studying veterinary medicine. During the past year there were only 592.

The committee report also noted that OSU's 1924 Veterinary College enrollment was down to 69, having declined steadily since 1920.

Another perspective is offered by Dr. Schalk in his history of the OSU Veterinary College. Citing national graduate figures, he writes:

> For the five year period 1922–1926, the 12 colleges and schools of the continent averaged fewer than 12 graduates per school—which is less than 3 new veterinarians a year for each of the 48 states over a five year period.

Schalk also notes that in these years OSU did better than other schools, turning out a yearly average of 23 graduates. But with the continuing decline in enrollment this average could not be sustained; over the succeeding five years graduation classes averaged only 15 members.

It was a trying time for veterinary education; at OSU there even were suggestions that the Veterinary College be downgraded into a department of Veterinary Science. But by the final years of the decade, the worst was over; enrollments were again increasing. At the 1928 Annual Meeting of the OVMA, the report of the Progress and Education Committee noted a marked improvement in the situation:

> There are this year 245 freshman students in the veterinary colleges of this country, which is an increase of 51 over the previous year. The total number of students now is 747. Ohio State has the greatest increase this year over previous years of any of the other colleges. . . . There are several factors which may have influenced this increased attendance. The hog cholera outbreak of last fall may be responsible for attracting the attention to the real need for veterinarians.

Hog cholera doubtless was a factor, focusing attention on veterinary medicine in much the same manner as the outbreak of foot-and-mouth disease in 1914-15. But another, more important factor, was the response of the veterinary colleges themselves. Faced with change they also changed, responding to the decline of the horse by placing new emphasis on food-producing livestock and broadening the scope of veterinary education. Describing the latter development at OSU, Dr. Schalk notes:

> It was during these years that special courses in meat, milk and food inspection, as well as subjects relating to breeding problems, were embodied in the curriculum.... One of the major changes was to establish a department of Veterinary Preventive Medicine, previously a subject given only superficial consideration.

With responses like these the colleges staked out new territory for veterinary medicine. In the process they reawakened the interest of potential students, saved themselves, and assured a vital continuing role for a profession which had begun the decade with its future in doubt.

Veterinary education was markedly changed by the events which spilled from the late teens into the 1920s. And so was veterinary practice. The victory of the internal combustion engine over the horse, the farm depression, and later the Great Depression all struck with equal force at the individual practitioner, who suddenly faced challenges every bit as unnerving as those confronting the veterinary colleges.

When the horse ceased to be a means of transportation, it also ceased to be for many veterinarians a means of livelihood. Hardest hit immediately were urban practitioners, many of whom depended on regular contracts with business firms maintaining large stables of horses. With the precipitous decline of the city workhorse, these veterinarians experienced not only a sizable loss of income but a real threat to their professional lives.

On the farms the workhorse prevailed longer and rural veterinarians still could count on some equine practice. But with the farm depression and, in 1929, the general economic collapse, many rural practitioners also fell on hard times. Farmers could no longer afford to care for their livestock and since a call to the vet meant spending money they didn't have, they didn't make the call.

Confronted by shrinking practices, these veterinarians, both urban and rural, also had to meet change by changing themselves. And for many the answer was to enter a hitherto peripheral area of veterinary medicine. It was the field of small animal care.

It would be inaccurate to say that veterinary medicine "found" small animals when it "lost" the working

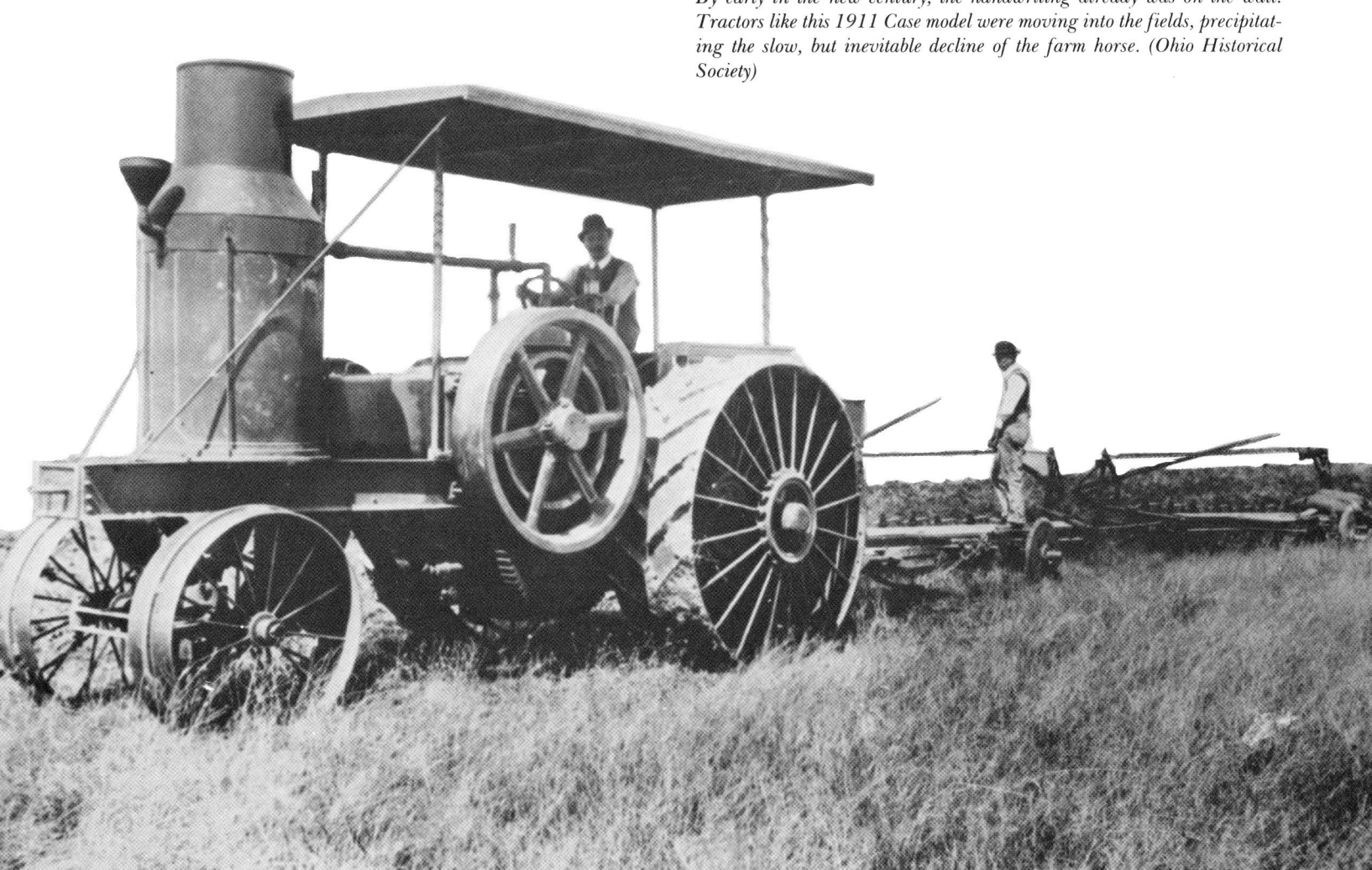

By early in the new century, the handwriting already was on the wall. Tractors like this 1911 Case model were moving into the fields, precipitating the slow, but inevitable decline of the farm horse. (Ohio Historical Society)

horse. Or that the depression-plagued 1920s created small animal practice. Actually, pet care (notably that of dogs) figured in veterinary practice from the beginning; as early as the 1840s the Englishman William Youatt wrote a veterinary medical text *The Dog* and the American edition in 1848 was the first comprehensive book on canine medicine published in the United States. In 1850, Dr. George Dodd included a section on canine disease in his book *American Cattle Doctor* and an 1879 Ohio publication by Dr. J.W. Johnson offering "the blessings of Homoeopathy" to "the irrational brute" had a six-page chapter on dog diseases. The chapter, incidentally, was only two pages shorter than a section dealing with the diseases of hogs.

But while small animal care was a part of veterinary practice in the latter half of the 1800s, it was definitely a secondary interest; the major focus of practitioners and veterinary educators alike was large animal medicine. This situation prevailed into the first decades of the 1900s. Dr. David Drenan, writing on *The Growth and Development of Small Animal Care* in the *Journal of the AVMA*, notes that in this period "the veterinary profession was still very reluctant to involve itself in this avenue of the profession."

So progress was slow; in the world of veterinary medicine, dogs, cats, and other "creatures small" remained second class citizens. While there were small animal practitioners and small animal courses at veterinary colleges, the field was not part of the mainstream of professional development.

With the 1920s, however, things began to change. In part, this was the result of changing public attitudes; pets were gaining wider acceptance and people wanted veterinary services. This trend was noted at the 1920 OVMA Annual Meeting when Dr. A. E. Cunningham presented an illustrated lecture on small animal hospitals, one of the first such presentations at an Association meeting. Commenting on public attitudes, Dr. Cunningham told his colleagues:

> With the development of our profession, higher standards of efficiency are being enforced and improvement in service demanded. . . . In recent years pets are receiving more and more attention and owners are demanding the best care possible . . .

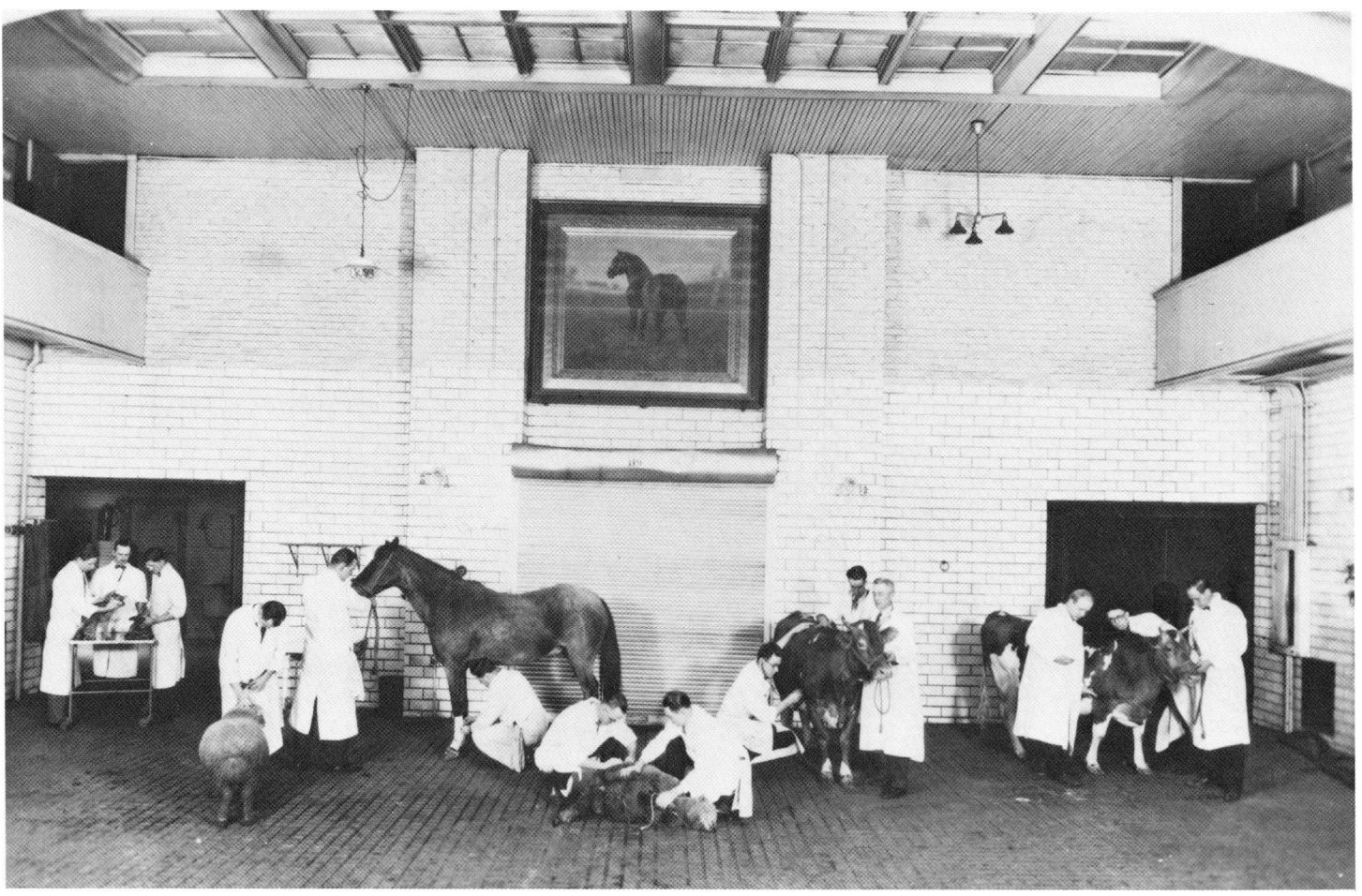

With the decline of the horse, veterinary colleges began to place greater emphasis on other livestock. The broadening of veterinary education is reflected in this obviously posed 1926 photo of activity in the Veterinary Clinic at OSU. (Photo Archives, Ohio State University)

The profession responded to this demand, as well as to other social and economic changes militating in favor of increased small animal practice. As already noted, prominent among the latter were the decline of the horse and the agricultural and general depressions which forced many veterinarians to shift to the small animal field to preserve their practices.

Reflecting the changing scene, the AVMA in 1923 had its first session devoted to small animal topics. The following year a small animal program was held, even though it took close to 300 letters to secure enough papers to round it out. And, in 1926, the national association featured the first section on small animal medicine.

Veterinary colleges also began responding to the increased emphasis on pet care, expanding their courses of study and accelerating research programs. OSU was a leader in this field; as early as 1911 the Veterinary College included a small animal wing in its new clinic building, perhaps prescient recognition of changes to come. And in 1921 OSU Professor O. V. Brumley, later dean of the Veterinary College, published his *Diseases of the Small Domestic Animals,* which for the next 30 years would be the "bible" of small animal medicine.

The expansion of small animal practice continued through the 1920s and into the succeeding decade. Growth was rapid and, inevitably, there were accompanying problems, including inadequate communication among small animal practitioners, limited information about animal hospital operations, and an absence of standards for small animal care. Concerned by the situation, progressive practitioners saw a need to bring some order to their field and their efforts resulted in a major achievement. It was the founding of the American Animal Hospital Association.

The AAHA was born in controversy. When small animal practitioners held a special session at the August, 1933 AVMA meeting to discuss common concerns and a possible organization, they attracted a sizable number of hostile colleagues, many of whom felt that the "dog doctors" were trying to take over the national association. The session was described as

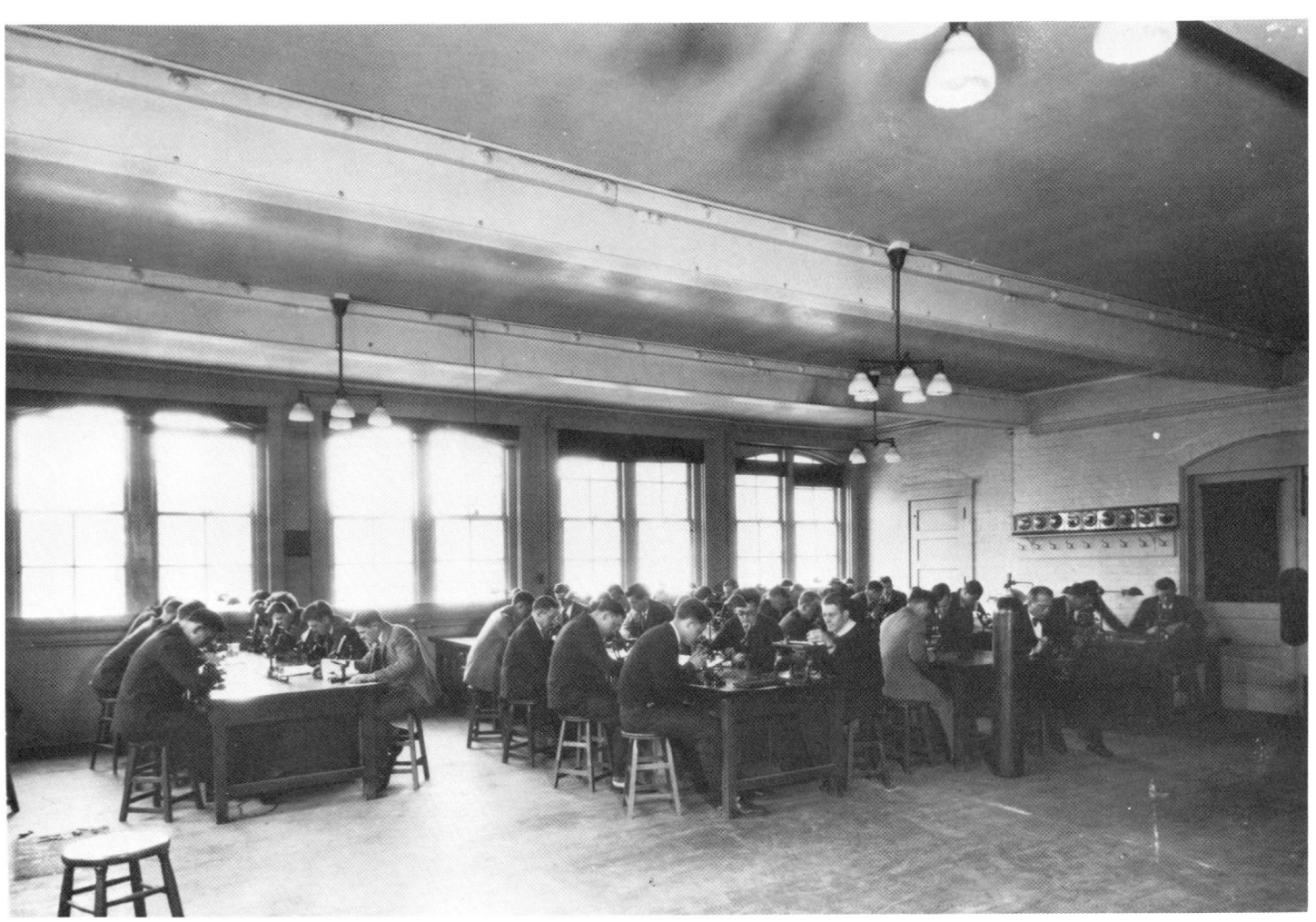

By 1931, when this picture was taken, veterinary enrollment at OSU was increasing. During the early and mid-1920s, the decline in enrollment was so serious there were suggestions that the College be downgraded to a department of Veterinary Science. (Photo Archives, Ohio State University)

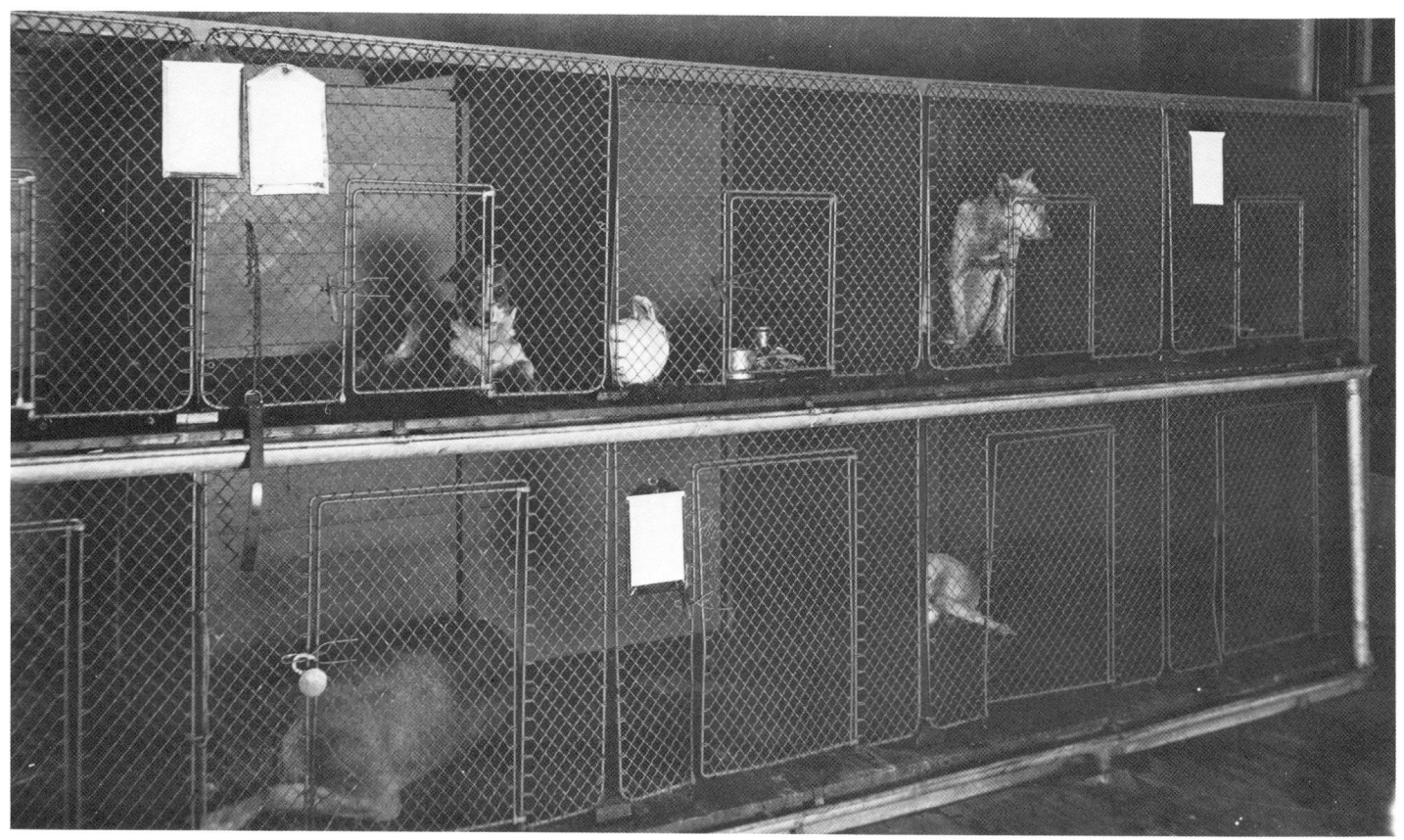

A section of the small animal wing in the Veterinary Clinic, 1915. The OSU college of Veterinary Medicine was an early leader in the field of small animal research and treatment. (Photo Archives, Ohio State University)

chaotic and produced no immediate results. But the groundwork was laid and, despite opposition, within three months the new organization was a reality.

One of its founders was Dr. Arthur C. Theobald of Cincinnati, a leader in small animal practice. In January 1934, he addressed the OVMA Annual Meeting, commenting on the first turbulent AVMA session and subsequent events:

> At the AVMA meeting in Chicago, we had a meeting which I'm sorry to say ended in chaos.... Before we left there, as I said before in chaos, we did appoint a chairman and a secretary. However, the chairman and secretary and some of the rest of us took it quite upon ourselves to start an organization. We met in November in the Palmer House in Chicago. We labored for two days and two nights in the formation of this new organization.

Dr. Theobald also told OVMA members that the founders of the AAHA "conscientiously believe that we're going in the right direction to form an organization of this kind" and history has proved him correct. Dr. Drenan, in his article on small animal care, suggests the founding of the AAHA was the greatest impetus to small animal medicine in the history of the profession and describes its standards for hospitals

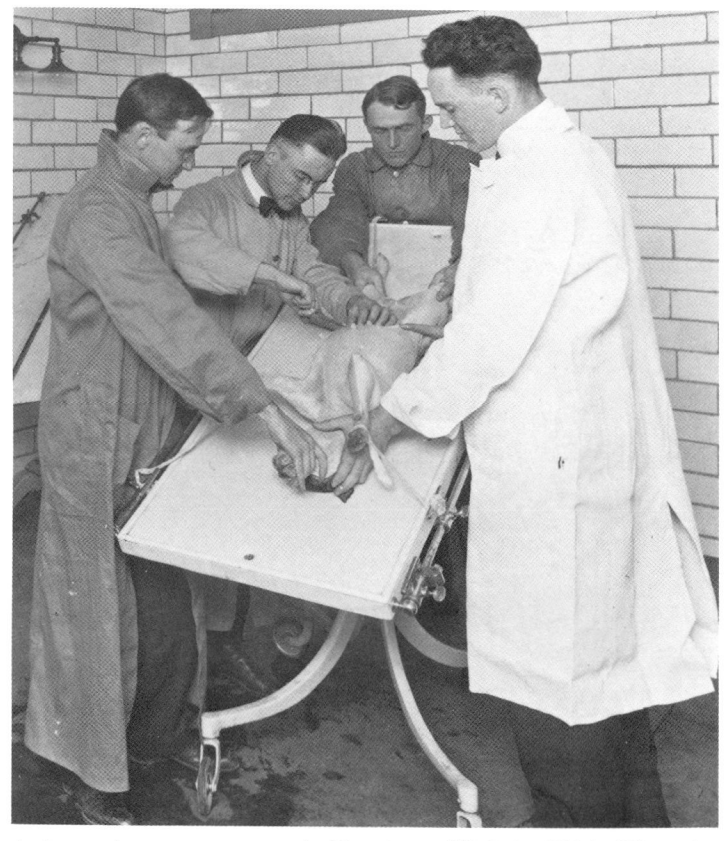

A dog undergoes surgery at the Veterinary Clinic in 1914. (Photo Archives, Ohio State University)

and equipment as "the greatest single force in the elevation of pet care facilities to this day."

It is important to note that the initial hostility to the AAHA did not last very long. In 1935, only two years after its founding, Dr. J.C. Flynn of Kansas City was elected president of the AVMA, becoming the first small animal practitioner to head the national organization.

With the success of the AAHA, small animal practice achieved a new level of maturity and recognition. Having shed its "poor relation" image, it continued to grow throughout the 1930s, buoyed by expanded small animal research and new disease treatments that increased the practitioner's effectiveness.

The small animal had arrived. And so had the small animal veterinarian.

For veterinary medicine the 1920s and 1930s were periods of trial, change and expanding horizons. In no area was this more evident than in the field of public health, where activities increasingly involved the professional veterinarian. A natural outgrowth of veterinary campaigns against epizootic diseases, the profession's role in public health work expanded over the years and was characterized by growing cooperation with human health practitioners, a trend which established a crucial alliance between the two health professions.

Veterinary involvement in public health concerns began early, paralleling the development of scientific veterinary medicine in the United States. One of the first major actions came in 1879 when the AVMA, alarmed by the animal plagues and epizootics which followed the Civil War, urged the establishment of a Veterinary Sanitary Bureau for the protection of both animal and human health. A year later, Dr. Frank Billings proposed creation of a Veterinary Sanitary Section in the National Board of Health and also urged establishment of a national veterinary institute. Billings, author of an early book dealing with the relation of animal diseases to human health, is credited by Dr. Calvin Schwabe with being the first to publicize "a well developed concept of veterinary activity in public health in the United States."

These efforts and others finally led to government action. The Bureau of Animal Industry was established as a division of the U.S. Department of Agriculture in 1884 and some two decades later the first federal meat inspection laws were passed. Both actions committed the government and veterinarians to important roles in the public health field.

In Ohio, the first recorded evidence of OVMA involvement in public health matters is in the Report of the 1915-16 Annual Meeting. It notes Association membership in the newly-formed Ohio Public Health

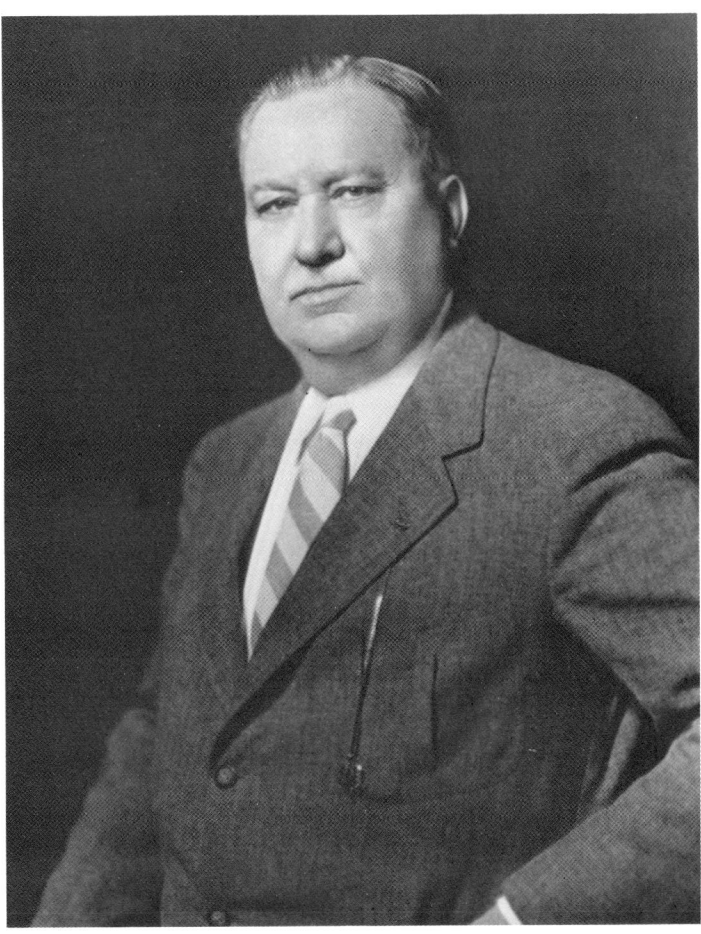

In 1921, Professor O. V. Brumley published his Diseases of the Small Domestic Animals, *the "bible" of small animal medicine. Professor Brumley later served as Dean of the College of Veterinary Medicine. (Photo Archives, Ohio State University)*

Federation, a group that also included, among others, the Ohio State Medical Association and the Ohio State Dental Society. Organized to "promote and systematize a Joint Campaign for the Conservation of Health in Ohio," the Federation was essentially a lobby group organized to support or oppose legislation relating to public health.

More direct professional activity was just ahead. This was the participation of Ohio veterinarians and the OVMA in disease control programs, a subject covered in a preceding chapter. The contributions of practitioners and the Association to this vital effort established the veterinary profession as a major force in the field of public health.

But not without some opposition. There was dissension in the veterinary ranks, a fact noted in the OVMA's 1970 History:

> The role of the veterinarian in public health was a very controversial one during the 1920s. There were those who felt that members of our profession, about 80 percent of whom were dependent upon agriculture and the livestock industry for

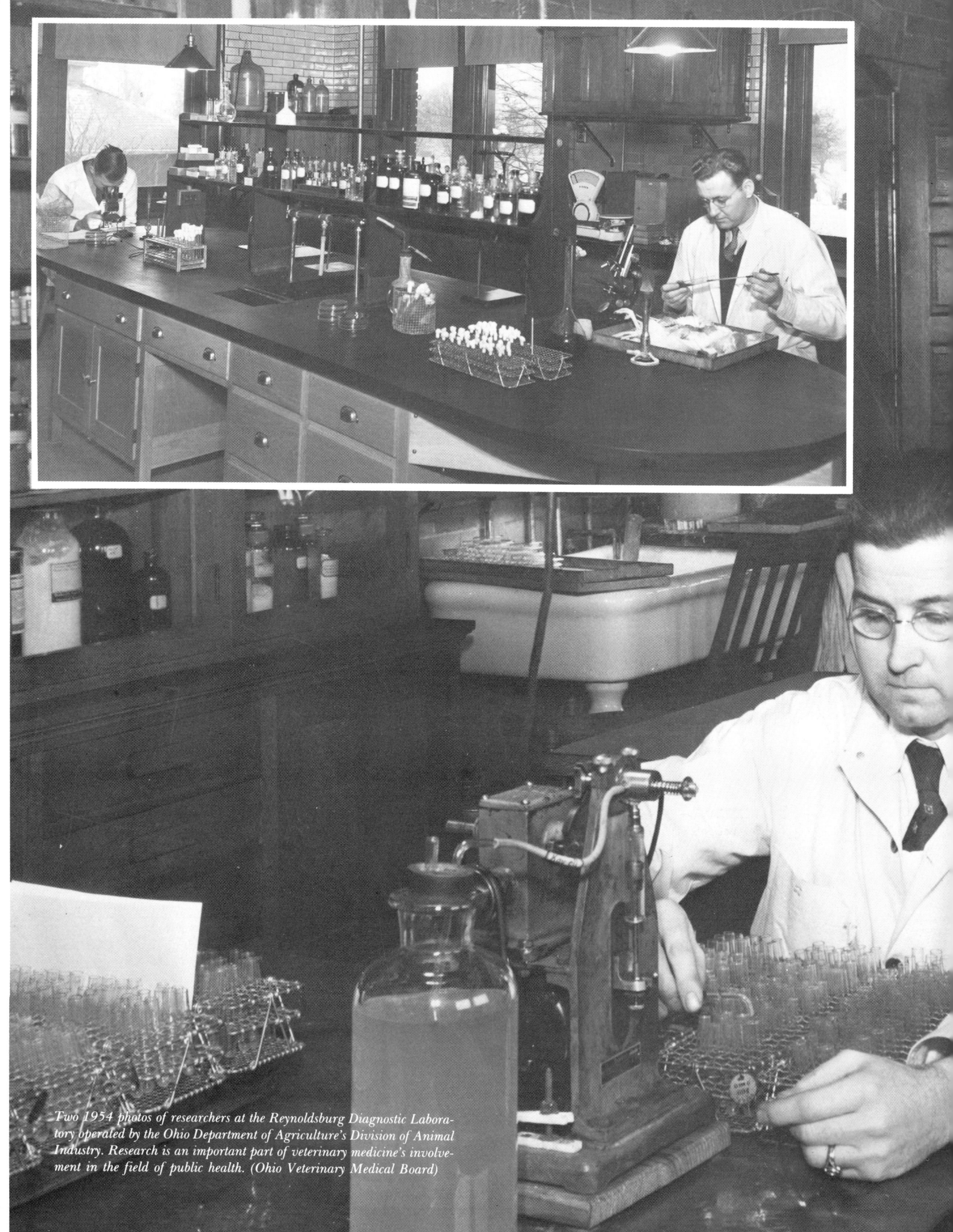

Two 1954 photos of researchers at the Reynoldsburg Diagnostic Laboratory operated by the Ohio Department of Agriculture's Division of Animal Industry. Research is an important part of veterinary medicine's involvement in the field of public health. (Ohio Veterinary Medical Board)

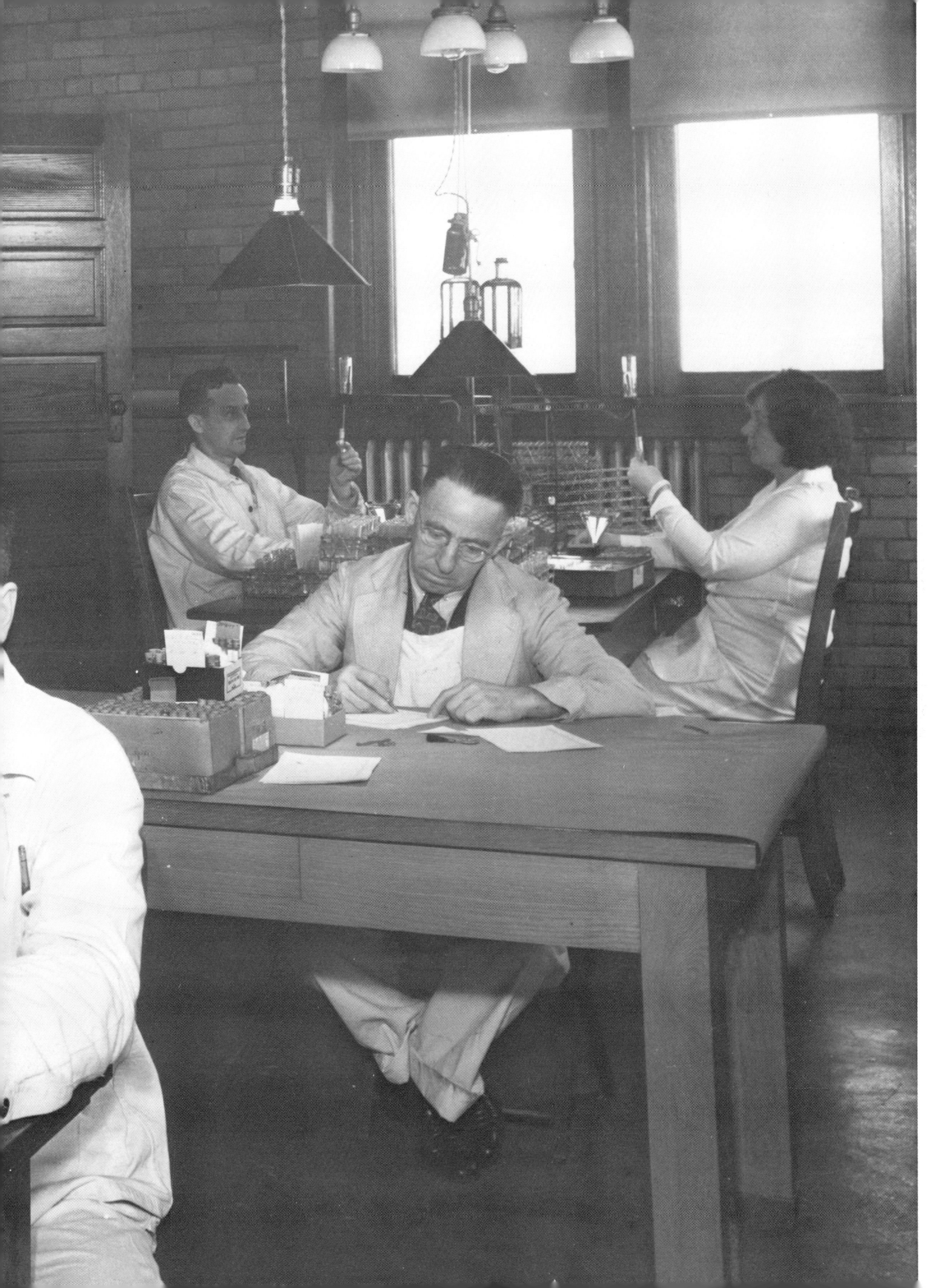

their livelihood, should not become involved in a matter of informing the public of the dangers of animal diseases, such as tuberculosis, undulant fever, etc., to the consuming public. On the other hand there were those who contended that where the public welfare is at stake, our profession and each of its members has a responsibility to so inform the public if we are to fulfill our true professional stature; we should do all in our power to assure public protection by obtaining their support for eradication of diseases and proper inspection of animal products to insure their wholesomeness.

The proponents of involvement prevailed. Veterinary medicine committed itself to assuring "public protection." And out of this commitment and the results that followed came even greater professional stature. On October 3, 1932, the *Ohio State Journal* editorialized:

> When three young women from other states registered as students in the college of veterinary medicine at Ohio State University, their action attracted attention to an important profession that has never been crowded and today hardly has enough skilled practitioners available to meet public needs. Scientific progress and changed conditions in the world have moved the skilled veterinarian far away from the old time horse doctor stage, and given him an important work in protecting public health in the homes, making him a valuable friend and servant of humanity.... Not only has the profession put under control the plagues and epidemics among animals... but it stands guard over much of the food that goes to family tables in the homes.

In succeeding years the "important work" of veterinarians continued to increase in significance. Their progress is perhaps best reflected in selected excerpts from the Annual Meeting reports of the OVMA Public Health Committee, which was established in 1931:

> *1939:* "In Ohio, the cities of Cleveland, Toledo, Akron, Youngstown, Canton, Columbus, Dayton, Marion, Sandusky, Ashtabula, Middletown, Massillon, Hamilton and Springfield are among those employing a number of veterinarians in Public Health work.

> *1949:* "In accordance with the growing importance of animal-borne diseases in the public health field, the Ohio Department of Health, in February 1948, added to the staff of its Division of Communicable Diseases, a public health veterinarian to study animal-borne diseases and institute programs for their control... it may be expected that the Ohio Department of Health will show increased activity in the field of animal diseases during the coming year.

> *1951:* "On October 30, 1950, in conjunction with the American Public Health Association, a one-day meeting, the Conference of Public Health Veterinarians, was attended by one member of this (OVMA) committee.... This conference shows more and more the importance that is being placed upon veterinary service in public health work.... Along the same lines and perhaps with broader objectives is a new development and *the first of its kind in the United States.* At the 1950 meeting of the Ohio Public Health Association there was organized a section on veterinary *preventive* medicine and public health.... The committee feels this to be a definite step forward in public health...

In 1969, there was further recognition of the importance of veterinarians in the public health field. On the recommendation of the OVMA, Dr. Bruce Wenger was appointed by the Governor as the first veterinarian to serve on the Ohio Public Health Council. And, in 1979, the Ohio Health Director, Dr. John Ackerman, announced establishment of an Advisory Committee to the Health Department's Veterinary Public Health program. In naming eight veterinarians to the committee, Dr. Ackerman noted:

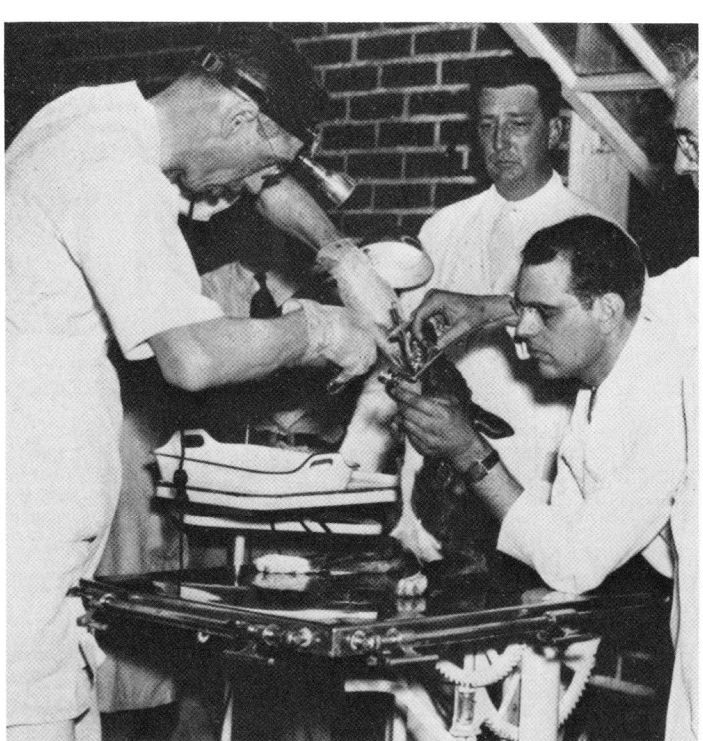

Ohio's first canine tonsillectomy, performed in 1931 at an OVMA meeting on the Ohio State Fair grounds. The three men in the center are Dr. Ashcraft of the OSU Veterinary College, Dr. Morgan Bates (then a senior student) and Dr. John F. Planz of Akron. (Photo: Dr. Morgan Bates)

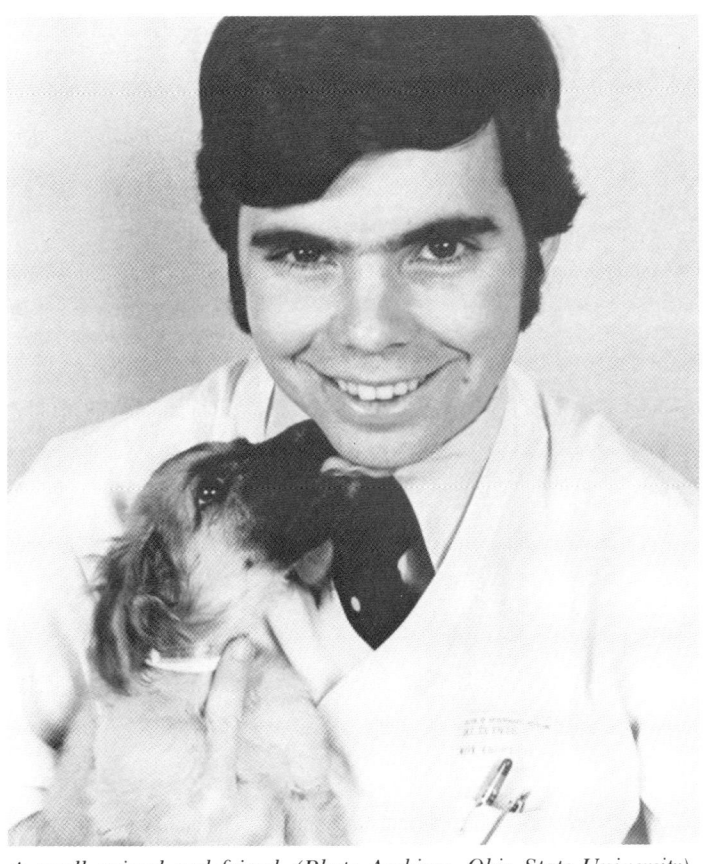

A small animal and friend. (Photo Archives, Ohio State University)

The contributions of the veterinary practitioner as part of the Health Team are significant.... The maintenance of an adequate supply of wholesome and nutritious food and the surveillance and control of zoonoses in companion animals in this age of rapid worldwide transportation demands an awareness beyond the capabilities of any government agency. The Department is aware of and will be responsive to problems at the grass-roots level, and the Committee fills that particular need.

Today, veterinary medicine is an integral part of the public health field in Ohio. In addition to the veterinarians employed by public health agencies, over thirty practitioners serve on community Boards of Health and another nine veterinarians are serving as Public Health Commissioners. Although marked on occasion by opposition, both internal and external, the profession's expansion into this field has been steady and its contributions to the public welfare of immense value.

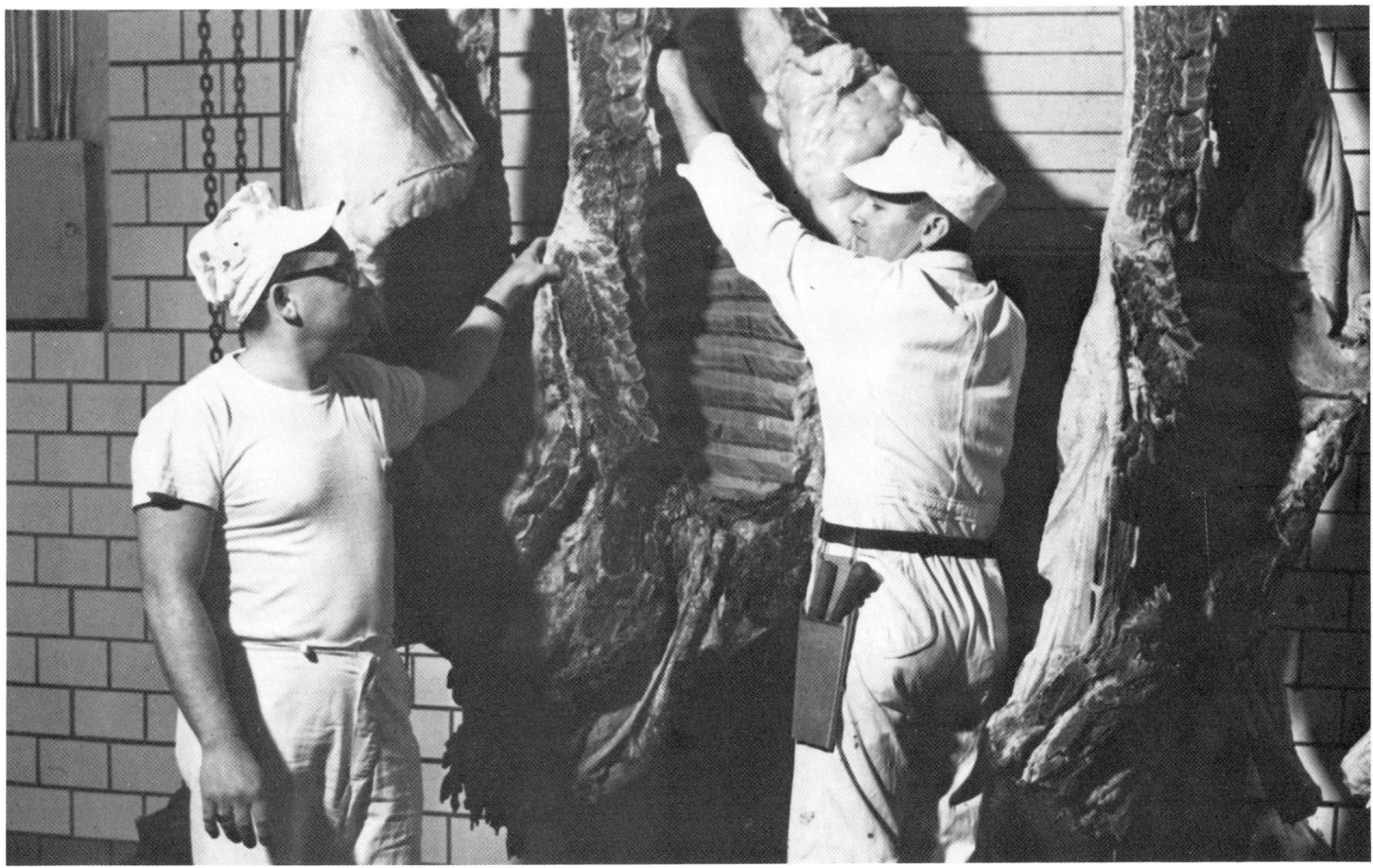

Meat inspection, another important public health responsibility of veterinary medicine. (Photo Archives, Ohio State University)

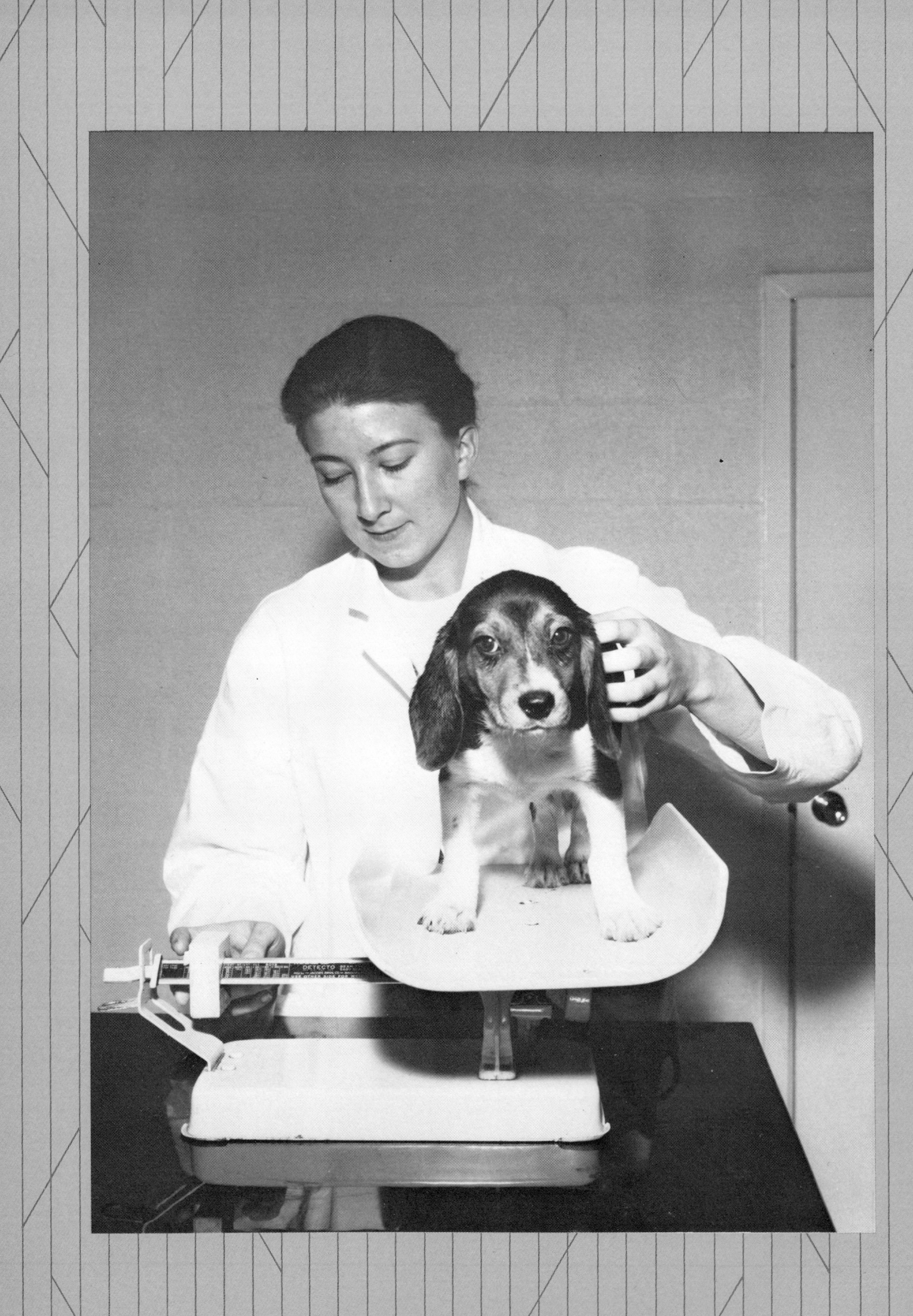

CHAPTER VI

POST WAR:
EXPANSION AND NEW DIRECTIONS

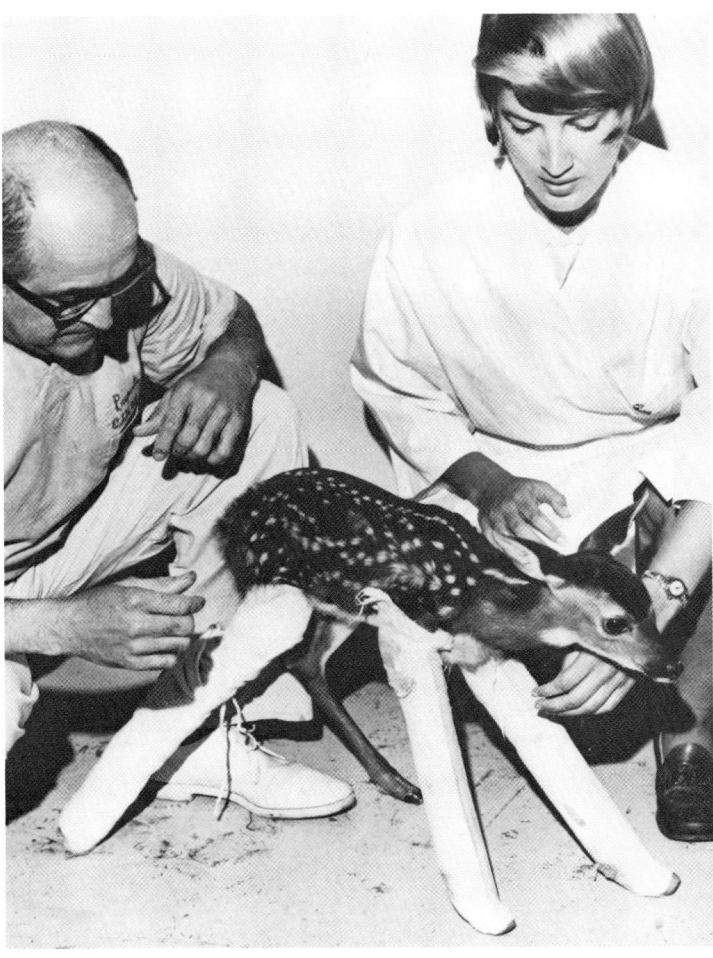

Wild animals can have their day with the veterinary, too, and this fawn needed more than one appointment. Today, wildlife management and related fields offer new opportunities for the veterinarian. (Photo Archives, Ohio State University)

> Immediately following ... World War II, the veterinary schools and colleges were confronted with a veritable flood of applicants.... (Among the reasons for this) may be cited the livestock industry demanding more veterinary service, a definite shortage of veterinarians, better compensation for veterinarians, and the G.I. Bill which assured financial support.... To meet this surge, OSU allowed a 35 percent increase in freshman enrollment.

This quote from Dr. Schalk's history of the OSU Veterinary College sums up the postwar picture of veterinary medicine. There was a surge of interest in the profession which set the stage for a new period of expansion.

The factors cited by Dr. Schalk were all valid reasons for the postwar boom. But there were others, too, the most important being the growing career opportunities offered by veterinary medicine, opportunities which continued to expand with the succeeding years.

Small animal care, now a major field of practice, sustained its momentum, with both disease treatment and preventive care becoming more sophisticated. A major advance came in the late 1940s with the introduction of penicillin, followed in the early 1950s by the advent of streptomycin and the broad spectrum antibiotics. Then, in the 1960s, there were other important developments in such fields as cardiology, ophthalmology and radiology. These advances, many resulting from stepped-up small animal research at veterinary colleges, accelerated the growth of small animal practice and made it an increasingly attractive field for veterinarians. Group hospitals developed and some veterinarians began to specialize in the care of individual species.

In this same period, the veterinary profession launched a campaign against the most-feared of all small animal diseases: rabies. Long a major threat to public health, rabies had stubbornly resisted eradication, largely because of the lack of any cohesive policy on vaccination. But a breakthrough finally came in 1946 when, at the urging of veterinarian Dr. Clinton Barrett, Summit County began a compulsory vaccination program. Three years later, at the 1949 OVMA Annual Meeting, Dr. Barrett reported on the results:

> Twenty-three percent of all the rabies in Ohio came from Summit County.... We passed regulations requiring compulsory vaccination in the spring of 1946. The record shows now that in 1945 and 1946 there were 227 cases in the county, and in 1947 and 1948 there were two

Small animal care became a major field of practice and continued to expand in the postware years, with both research and treatment becoming more sophisticated. (Photo Archives, Ohio State University)

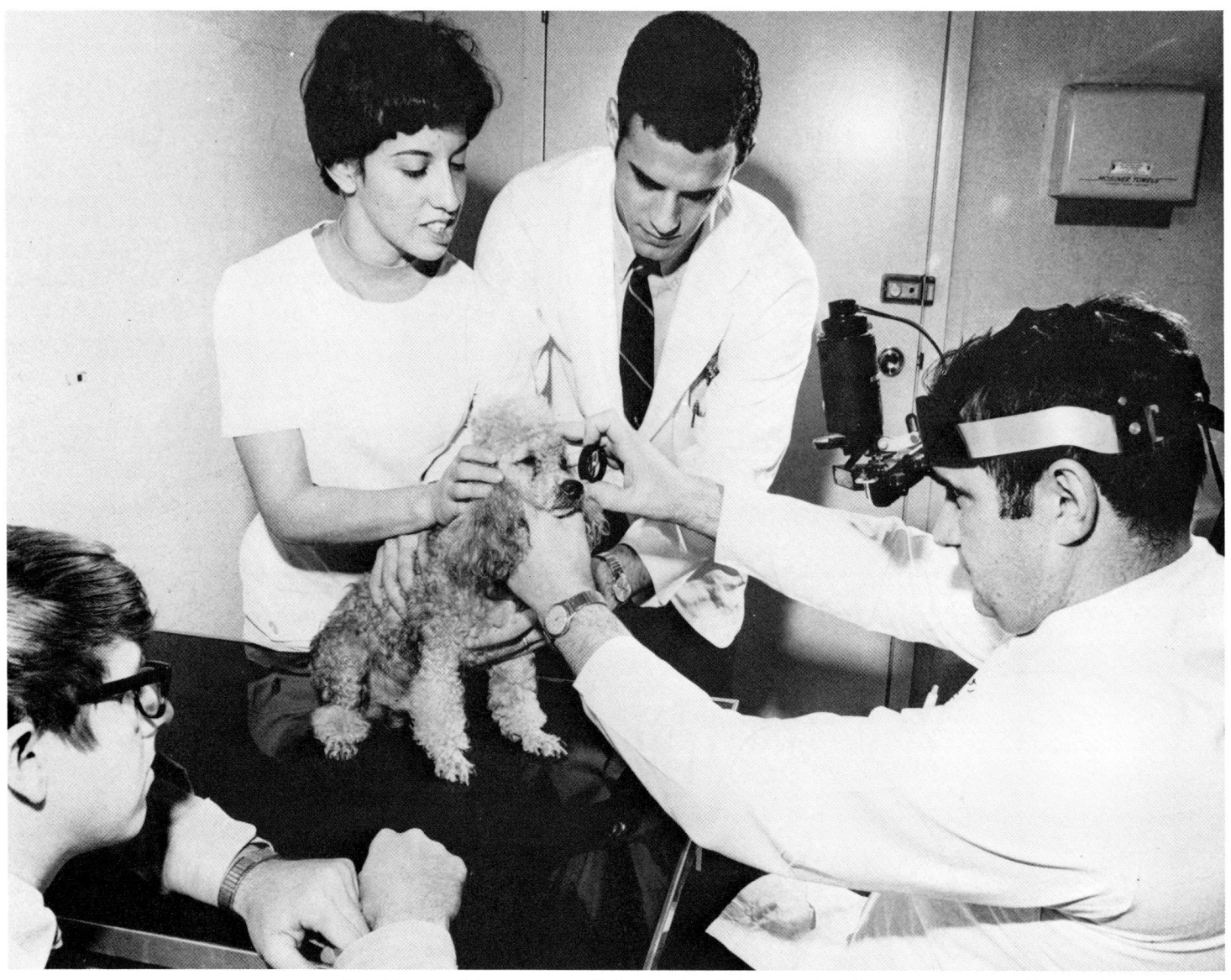
Developments during the 1960s in such fields as ophthamology, cardiology and radiology resulted from stepped-up small animal research and accelerated the growth of small animal practice. (Photo Archives, Ohio State University)

cases. So it is not a question of the efficiency or the adequacy of vaccination programs in a locality; it is just how far the control measure should go.

At the same meeting, similar success was reported by Hamilton County, which initiated a compulsory vaccination program in 1948. Twenty thousand dogs were vaccinated and over the next year not a single case of rabies was reported.

The experiences of Summit and Hamilton counties proved conclusively that compulsory vaccination worked and in succeeding years many other counties and communities followed their lead. Ohio had its last major rabies outbreak in 1959–60; by 1977 the incidence of the disease was at an all-time low and although there was an increase in cases in 1982, they were confined to wild animals (25 skunks, 1 fox, 1 bat) and two cows. The days when, as one veterinarian put it, "people bitten by a dog didn't sleep very well" were fading.

Significantly, the successful campaign against rabies was the result of local initiative, not state action. Although the OVMA and public health authorities pressed periodically for state legislation mandating vaccination, none has ever cleared the Ohio General Assembly. That effort remains part of the unfinished agenda.

With rabies blunted as a serious threat to public health, the OVMA turned to another small animal problem, that of overpopulation. In May 1973, the Association newsletter announced formation of a task force to investigate Ohio's pet population "explosion" and a year later reported on an OVMA response to the problem:

Members of the OVMA will donate their time and skills to a surgical sterilization program for pets of low income families . . . income from the program will be donated to the non-profit Ohio Animal Health Foundation and will be used to support research in effective anti-fertility drugs. . . . Programs throughout the state will be conducted by local veterinary associations.

The sterilization program was developed by the OVMA's Task Force on Pet Overpopulation and the non-profit Foundation established by Association trustees. Under the plan, low income families were charged a minimum $20 fee for pet sterilization and then referred by local review committees to participating veterinarians with the fees being donated to the Foundation in the names of the veterinarians contributing their services. The sterilization program was the first of the Foundation projects; it later expanded fund-raising efforts and the scope of its small animal research interests. Between 1974 and 1980, it distributed over $22,000 in research grants to the OSU Veterinary College and other veterinary schools.

Paralleling postwar developments in the small animal field were changing conditions in the livestock industry. Livestock care was no longer the absolute monarch of veterinary medicine, but it remained a major area of involvement. Even as the campaigns against the epizootic diseases were winding down to a successful conclusion, economic trends in the livestock industry were creating a demand for new and more sophisticated forms of veterinary practice. This challenge to the profession was noted in an editorial in the November 1959 issue of the OVMA magazine *The Ohio Veterinarian:*

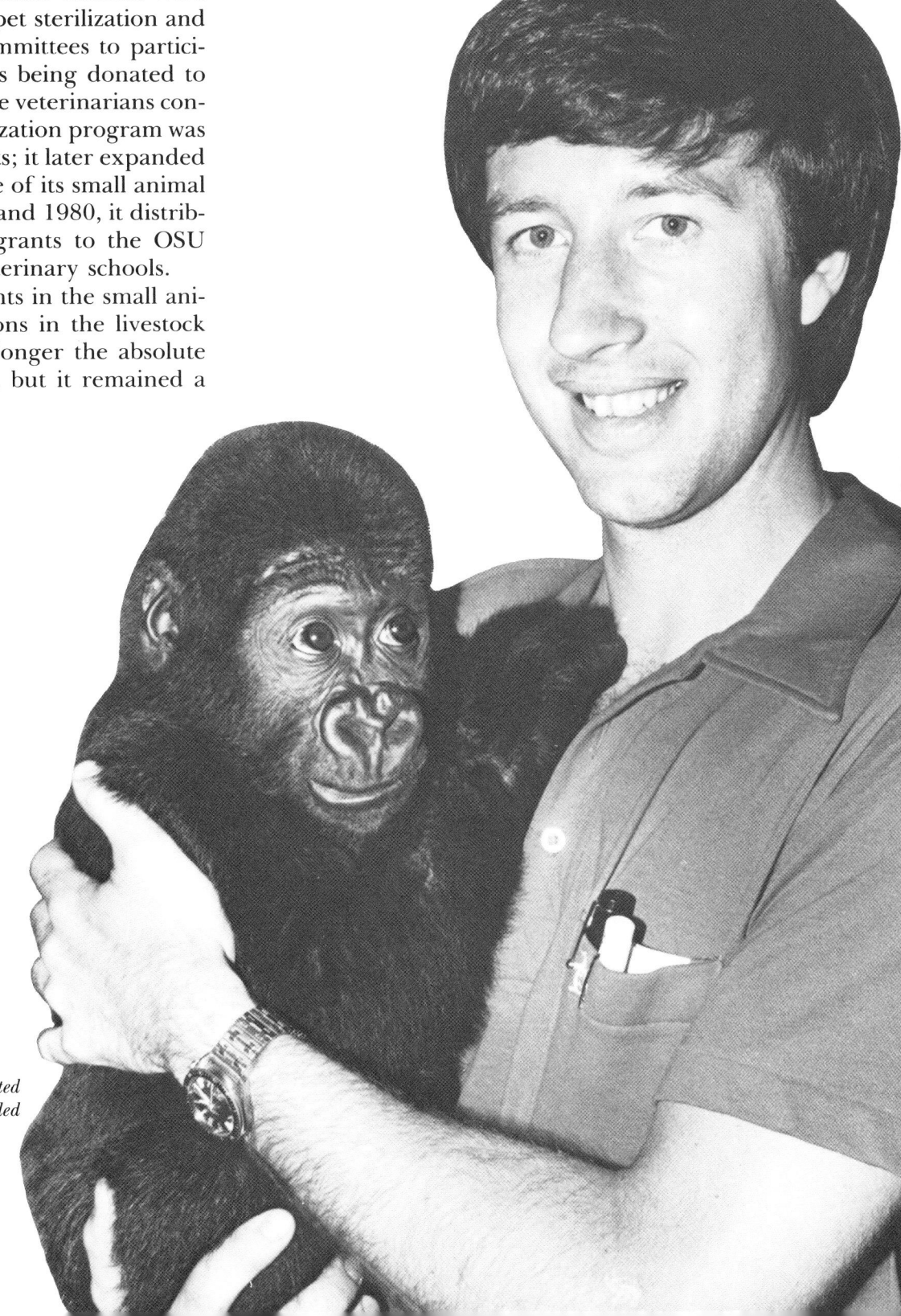

New career opportunities have also been created by the growing popularity of zoos and expanded efforts to preserve endangered species. (Photo, Cincinnati Zoo)

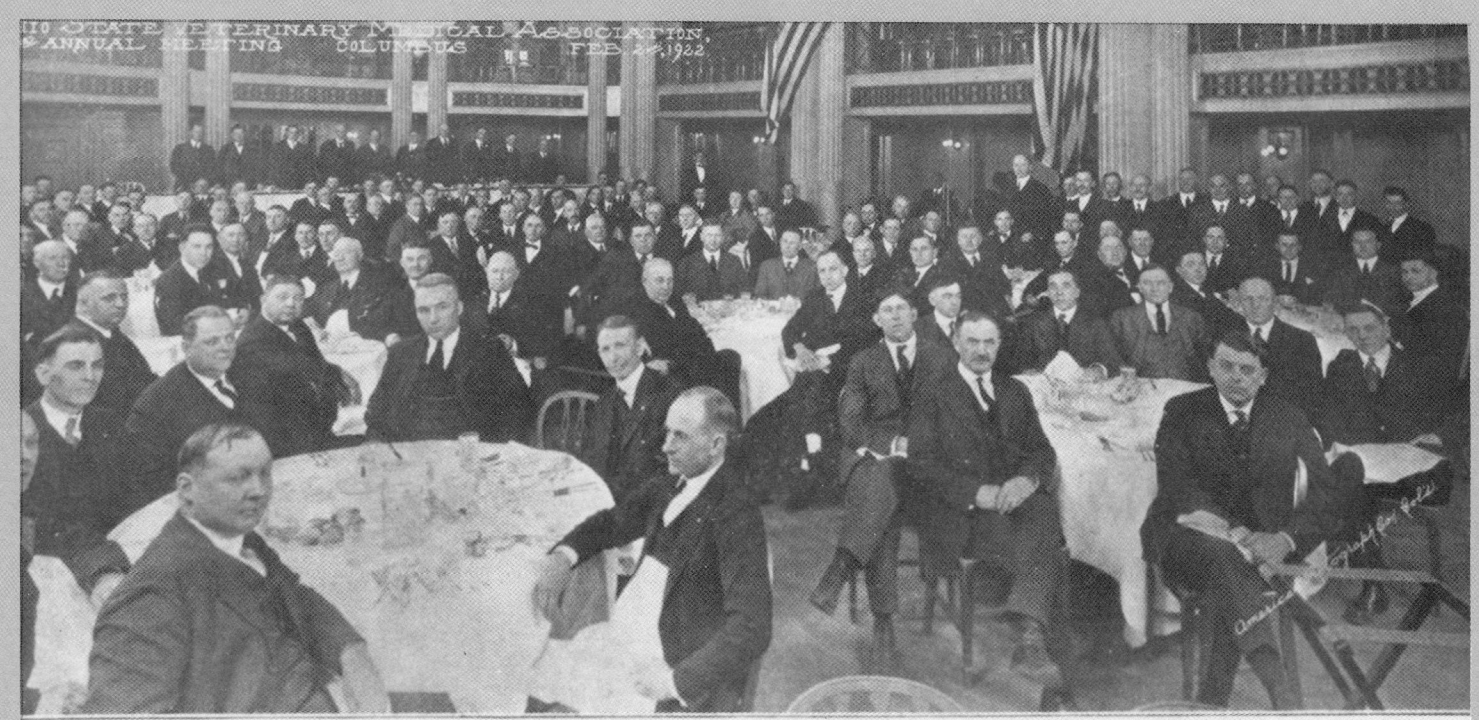

DINNER SESSION — HOTEL DESHLER

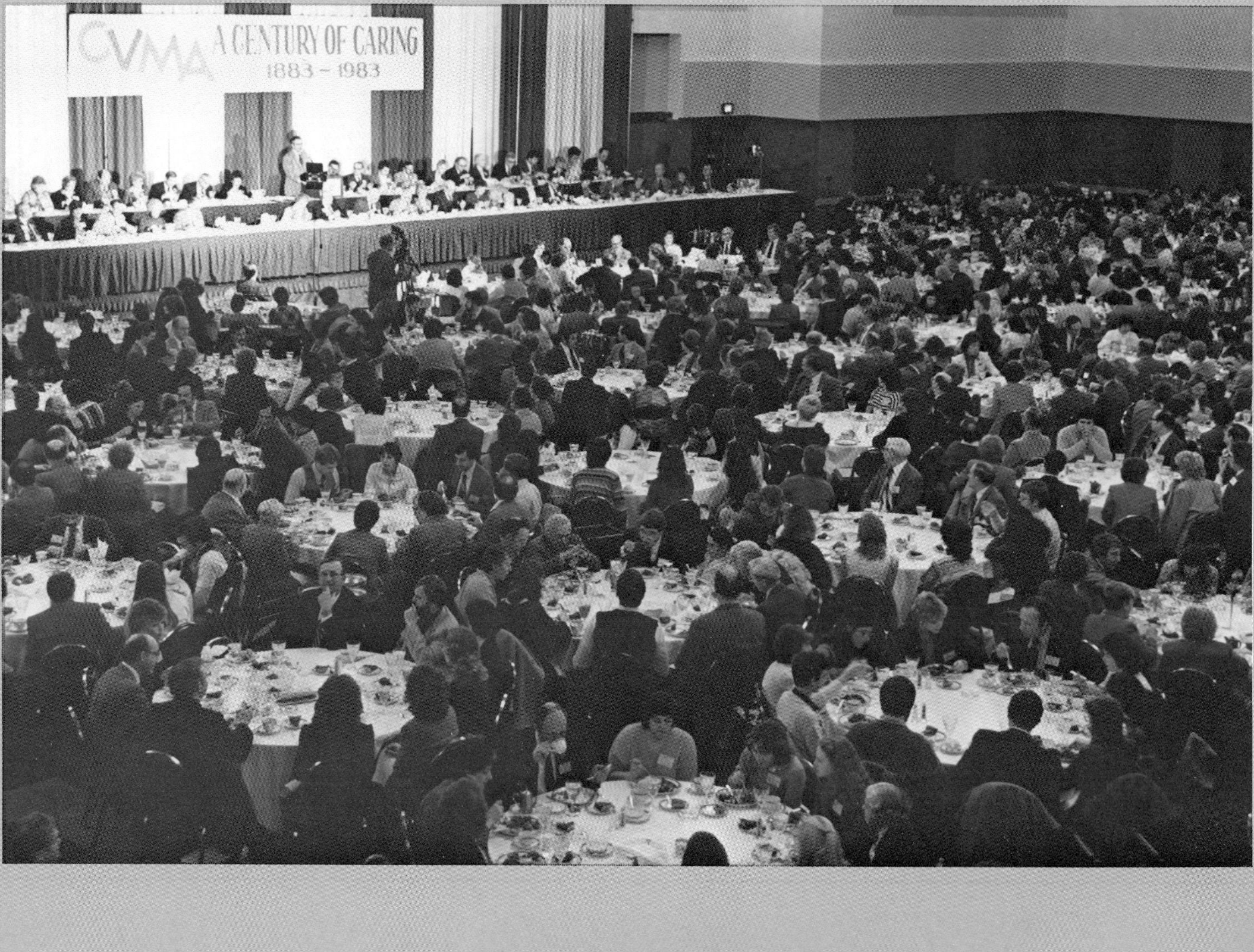

The time is past when 'the eye of the master' alone fattens his cattle. Livestock production is big business. Just like any manufacturing plant has a full-time maintenance crew to prevent breakdown, so also the livestock industry must maintain an operation to avoid breakdown. The veterinary profession must play a big part in this operation. This involves becoming familiar with the new nutritional advances, not only from the point of preventing disease, but also from the point of economics in the feeding operation which continuously is becoming more important.

In the same issue, this trend was discussed by Dr. Mervin G. Smith, Chairman of the OSU Department of Agricultural Economics. Writing on "vertical integration" and its impact on veterinary medicine, he observed:

> (Vertical integration is) the coordination of the management of the various stages of farm production, farm supply, processing and marketing or merchandising of agricultural products.... This may be a very important period or landmark in the history of agriculture.... We will have more vertical integration (and) veterinarians will be faced with new situations and problems.

Among the latter, Dr. Smith cited fewer farmers to serve, larger and more specialized farms, and the need to deal with "so-called integrators or managers of integrated systems." He also commented on the response that would be required from the veterinary profession:

> The veterinarian will need in some cases to offer a package of services, such as a scheduled program of preventive treatment and regular tests and examinations. Besides emergency calls, he may contract more services.... Since veterinarians will be dealing with larger specialized and yet varied business firms, they will need to know more about the agricultural businesses with which they are dealing.

This concept was not entirely new to veterinary medicine; a simpler version of it known as "herd health care" dated back at least to the 1920s. But in the postwar period of social and economic change, this approach to livestock care took on increased scope and complexity. Agriculture had always been "big business"; now more and more farmers were becoming "big businessmen" and the veterinary profession had to meet their expanding needs.

The OVMA Annual Meetings of 1922 and 1983, the latter launching the Centennial Year. In a single decade between 1971 and 1981, OVMA membership increased by 61 percent and topped 1,700 in 1983. (OVMA files)

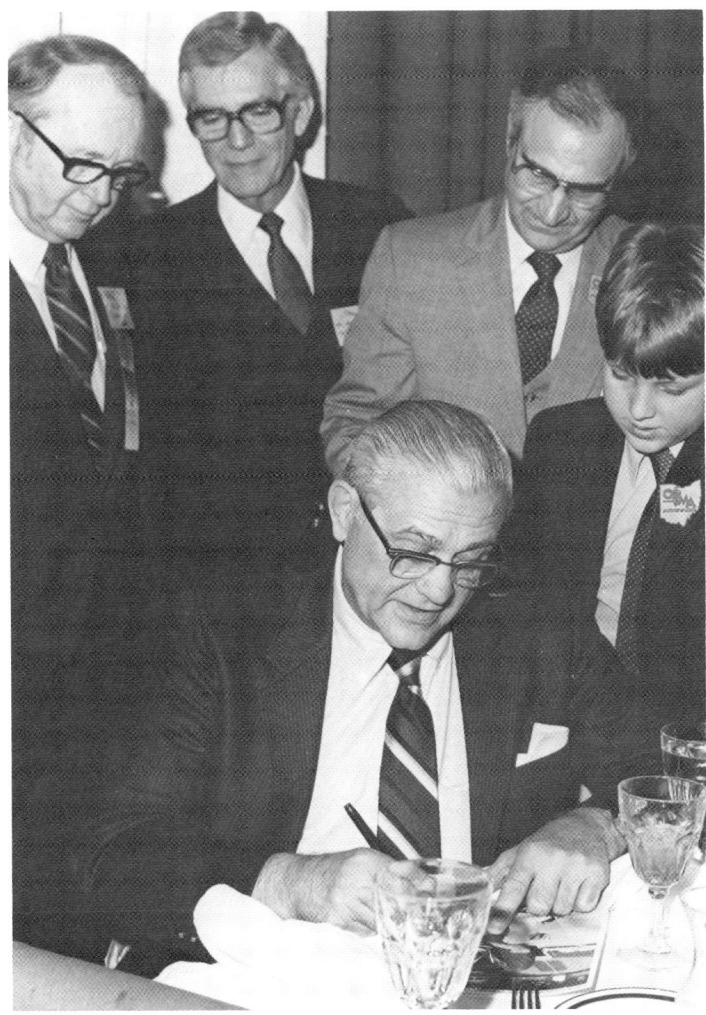

Woody Hayes, a frequent and popular guest at OVMA sessions, signing autographs at the 1983 Annual Meeting. (OVMA files)

It also had to meet an expanding demand for service in other areas, a key one being the field of medical research. As the veterinary profession evolved, the earlier, sometimes uneasy relationship between animal and human medicine was strengthened and the concept of "one medicine" gained increasingly wider acceptance. The new status of the veterinarian in medical research was noted by Dr. Walter R. Krill, Dean of the OSU Veterinary College, in *The Ohio Veterinarian* of June, 1960:

> While the animal health field is and will always remain the primary concern of the veterinary profession, there has been a growing realization on the part of those in the allied health fields as the role of veterinary science in the overall health program.... Since all biological research requires the use of animals, the demands for veterinarians to supervise animal colonies to insure the validity of research results and to participate as part of research programs are far beyond the supply of qualified personnel.... We can expect

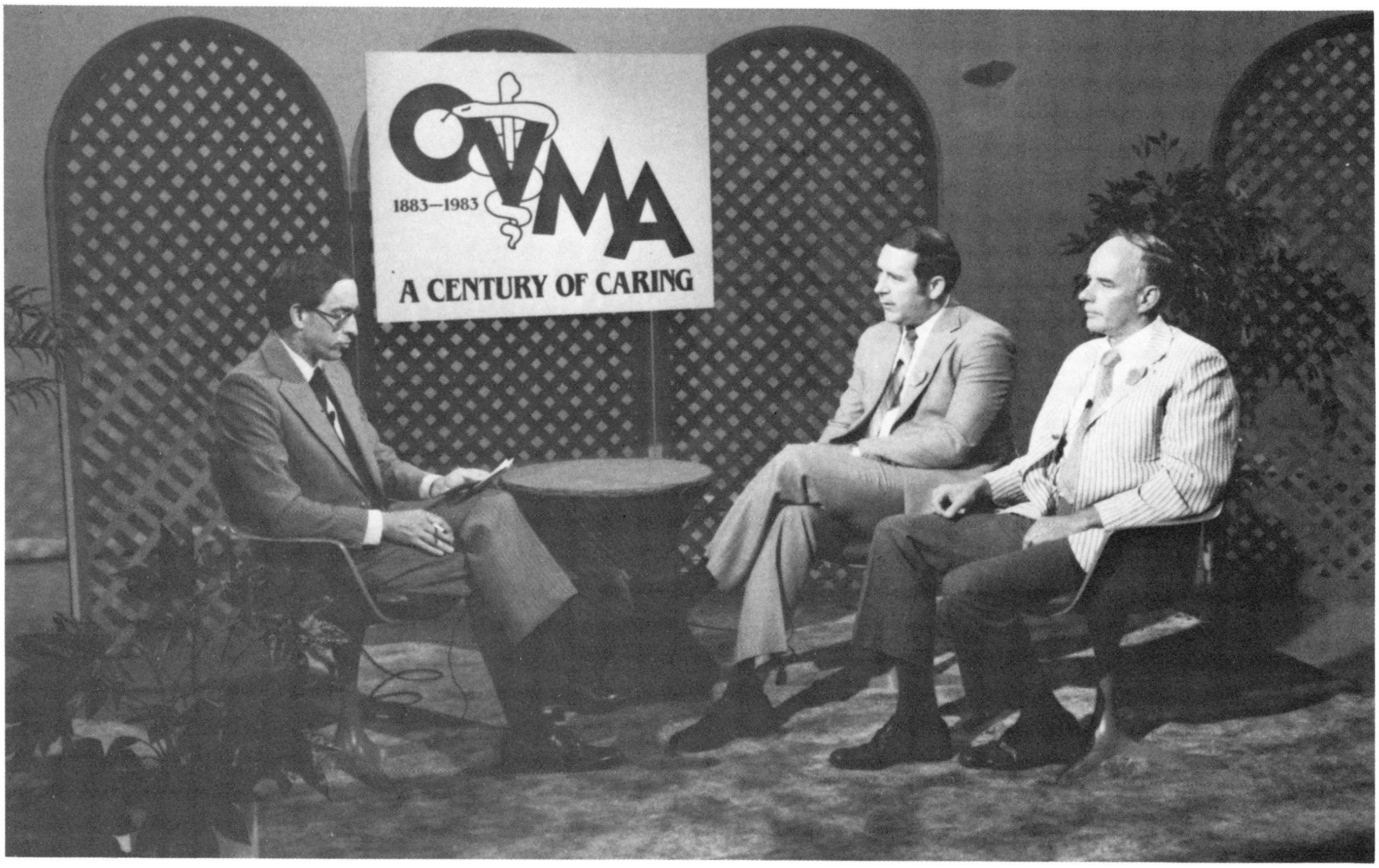

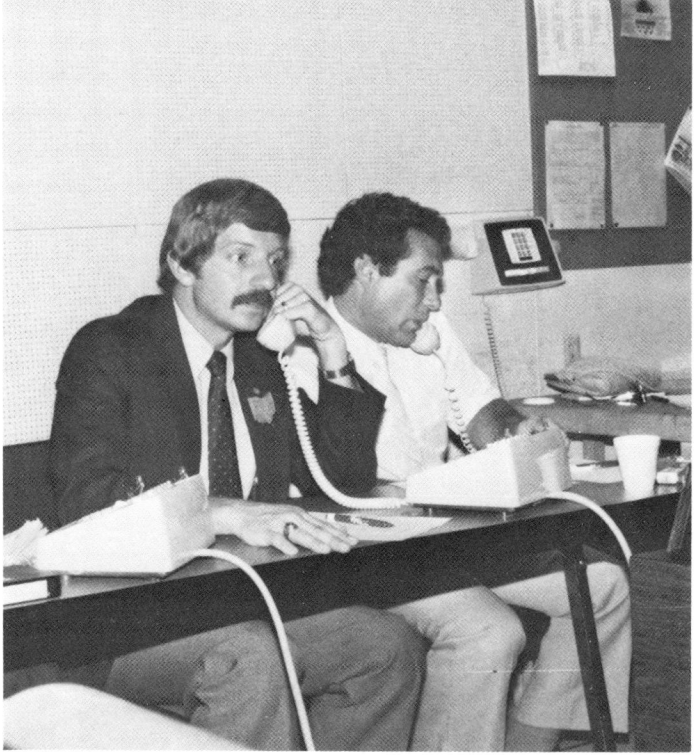

One of the most successful public information efforts of the 1983 Centennial Year was the statewide public television program "Ask Your Veterinarian," which gave viewers an opportunity to phone in questions about animal care. (OVMA files)

the demands for veterinarians in this field to increase in the years ahead.

Dr. Krill's prediction was borne out. In the ensuing years, veterinary participation in medical research continued to expand and today it is one of the most important responsibilities of the profession.

Another event of the postwar years deserves passing reference. While veterinary medicine was responding to new opportunities, it was also welcoming back an old friend and long-time sustainer, the horse. After reaching a low ebb in 1955, when there were only about 3 million horses and less than 100 equine practitioners in the country, the horse staged an amazing comeback, reemerging as a popular sport and recreational animal. The number of horses doubled between 1960 and 1970 and again between 1970 and 1980; today in Ohio there are more horses registered than at any time in the past. The result was a resurgence of equine practice and renewed emphasis on equine courses in the veterinary colleges.

In the 1970s, the veterinary profession itself initiated a change, this being a major revision of the Practice Act. A review by the OVMA of existing legislation began in 1971, but it was not until 1975 that the text of a proposed new act was completed. It embodied some significant new provisions, including:

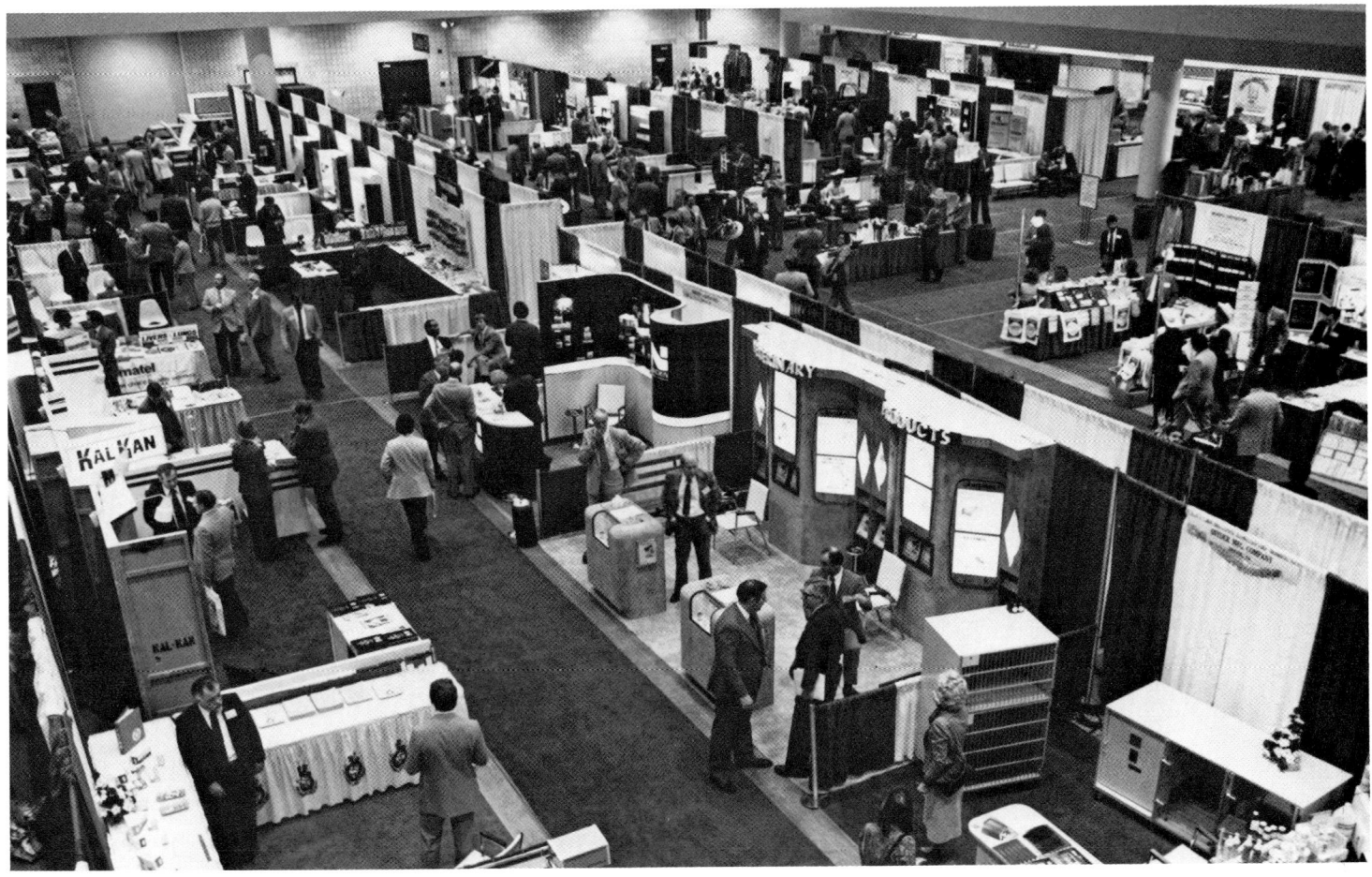
Another illustration of OVMA growth has been the steady increase in the number of exhibit booths at Annual Meetings. In 1983, over 120 booths were sold. The same year Annual Meeting attendance was over 3,000. (OVMA files)

First, ten hours annually of required continuing education, acceptable to the Ohio Veterinary Medical Board.

Second, the certification of animal technicians, and approval of either their formal training or experience by the Board.

Third, funding of the Board through an annual relicensing fee (for both veterinarians and animal technicians), in order to permit it to implement these duties.

The bill was sponsored by a veterinarian, State Representative Walter McClaskey, and passed both the House and the Senate. It was signed into law on July 18, 1975.

The new legislation was a milestone for veterinary medicine in Ohio; one veterinarian has described its passage "as the time when the profession reached maturity." In proposing new and more stringent standards and then guiding their passage into law, the OVMA dramatically demonstrated the profession's commitment to keep its own house in good order and further enhanced the status of the veterinary practitioner.

In addition, by requiring annual relicensing fees, the new Practice Act provided badly-needed funding for the State Veterinary Medical Board. And it brought under state regulation for the first time the growing number of animal technicians who served the profession in paraprofessional roles. The latter's status was now clarified; the Act defined a graduate animal technician as "A person who has received a degree in animal technology or a comparable degree from a school recognized by the Ohio Veterinary Medical Board and who is employed by and under the supervision of a licensed veterinarian." It also mandated for animal technicians "such reasonable continuing education requirements . . . as the Board may determine to be necessary." With this recognition and the setting of new standards for their profession, the status of animal technicians also was greatly enhanced.

The new Practice Act, with its emphasis on higher standards and continuing education, took on special significance in the years just ahead. Along with other professions (and institutions in general) veterinary medicine had to face increased public scrutiny as the consumer movement surfaced and grew, bringing

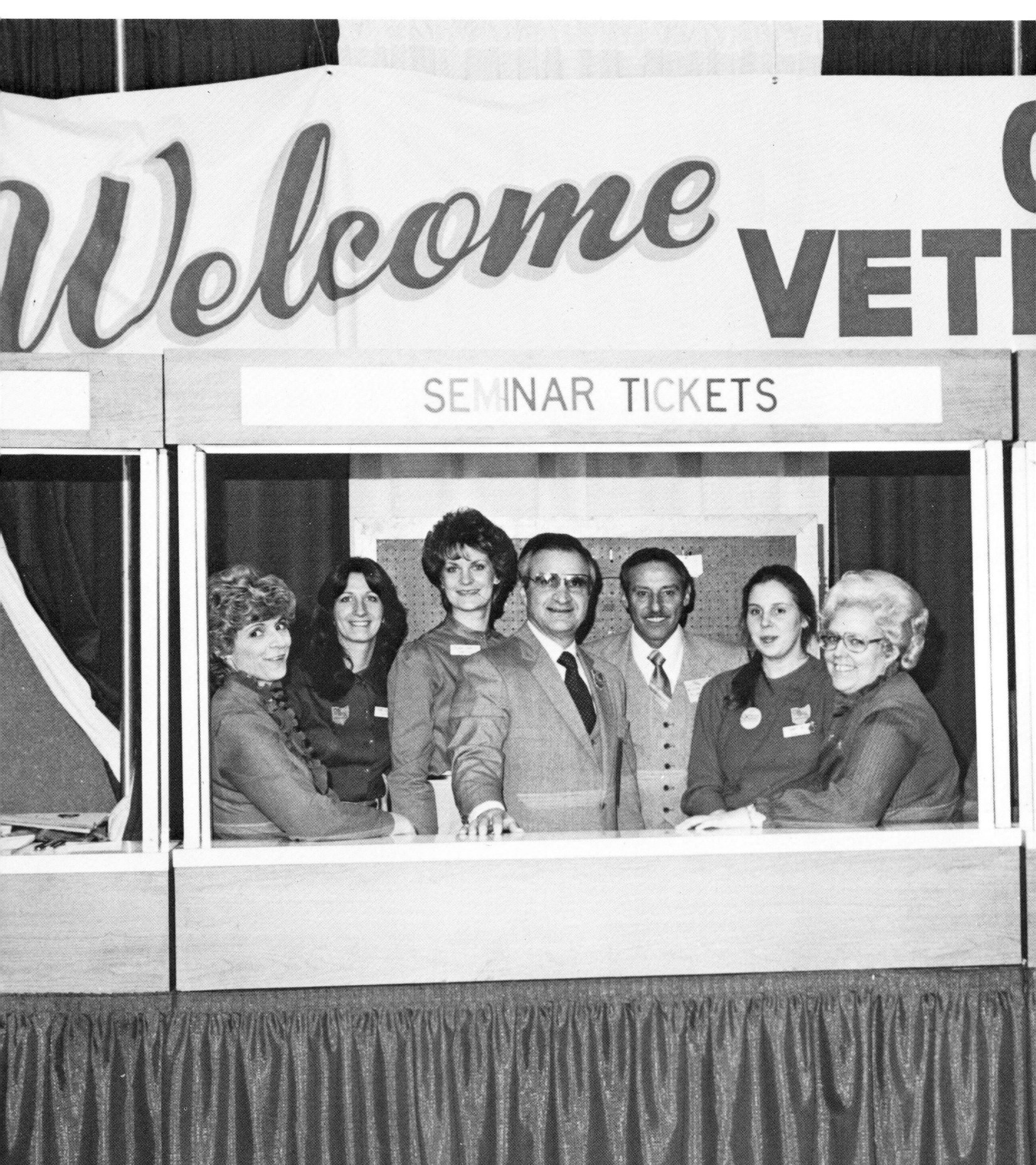

The welcoming committee at the 1983 Annual Meeting. (OVMA files)

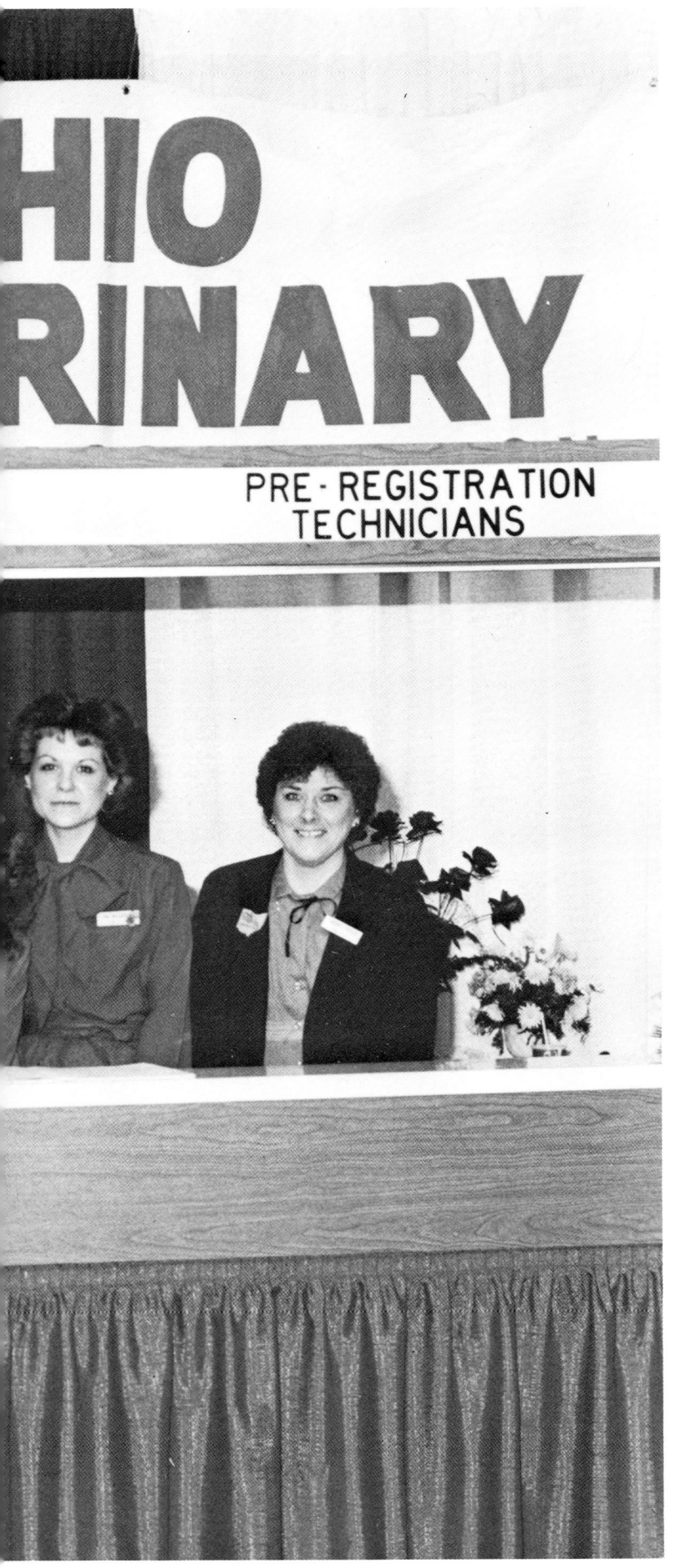

with it the threat of new government regulation. At the OVMA's 1977 Annual Meeting, Executive Secretary Gene P. King focused on this sharpened public sensitivity and the response it mandated:

> This professional Association must take action against those who do not meet the standards of offering professional services to the public.... The State Board of Veterinary Examiners (must) ... reassess their past history and develop a course of action which is responsive in assuring that the public's interest is maintained.... The action by the professional association and State Board is necessary or we will find ourselves in the hands of some other state agency which will totally dictate all our actions.... The public must know that we are willing to police our own ranks and that we are making an effort to see that the highest quality of veterinary care, at the most reasonable cost, is being offered.

In a very real sense, the new Veterinary Practice Act anticipated the rising concern for "consumer rights," with the result that the profession could deal with it from a position of strength when it became an issue. Coupled with continuing efforts to maintain high standards and protect the public interest, this voluntary initiative helped assure that veterinarians would remain the masters of their own profession.

In these years, as veterinary medicine and its practitioners continued to grow in stature, the OVMA itself experienced steady and impressive growth. Association membership topped the 1,000 mark in 1971; by 1976 it was close to 1,400, and by 1979 over 1,500. Two years later, at the 1981 Annual Meeting, Executive Secretary King commented on statistics reflecting a decade of growth:

> Those statistics reflect membership, a growth of 61 percent; they reflect the total expenditures for the association, a growth of 135 percent; they show attendance at our annual conventions, a growth of 95 percent; and they show the number of exhibit booths sold at this annual meeting, a growth of 45 percent.

And at the beginning of the 1983 Centennial Year, King could report:

> ... an annual income and expense of $375,000, over 120 exhibit booths sold, a total membership of 1,700 and attendance at the Annual Meeting of over 3,000.

The OVMA had come a long way since the turn of the century when, at the 1904 Annual Meeting, the Association reported 110 members, but only 45 of them current with their dues and, therefore, in good standing.

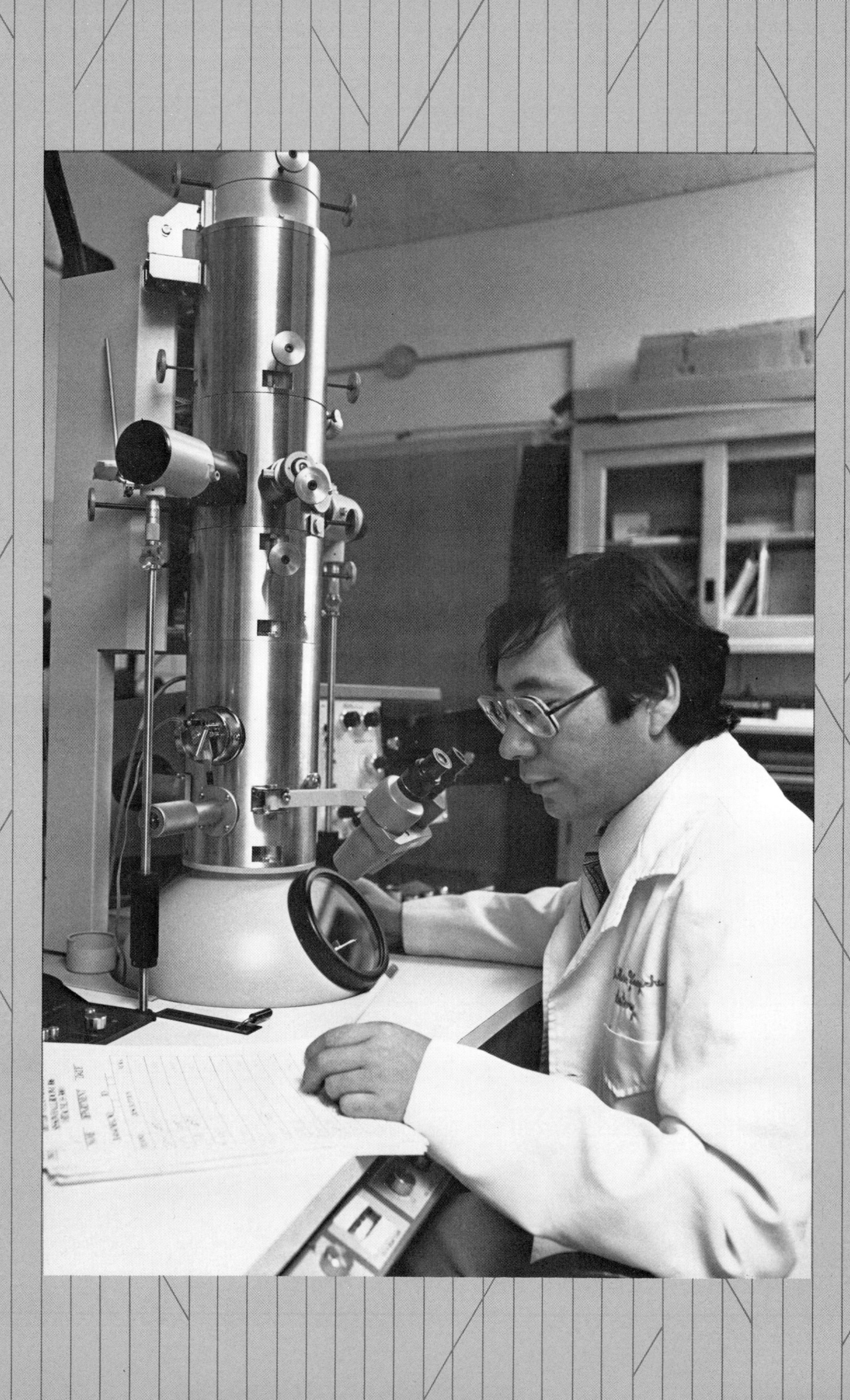

CHAPTER VII

OSU: THE LATER YEARS

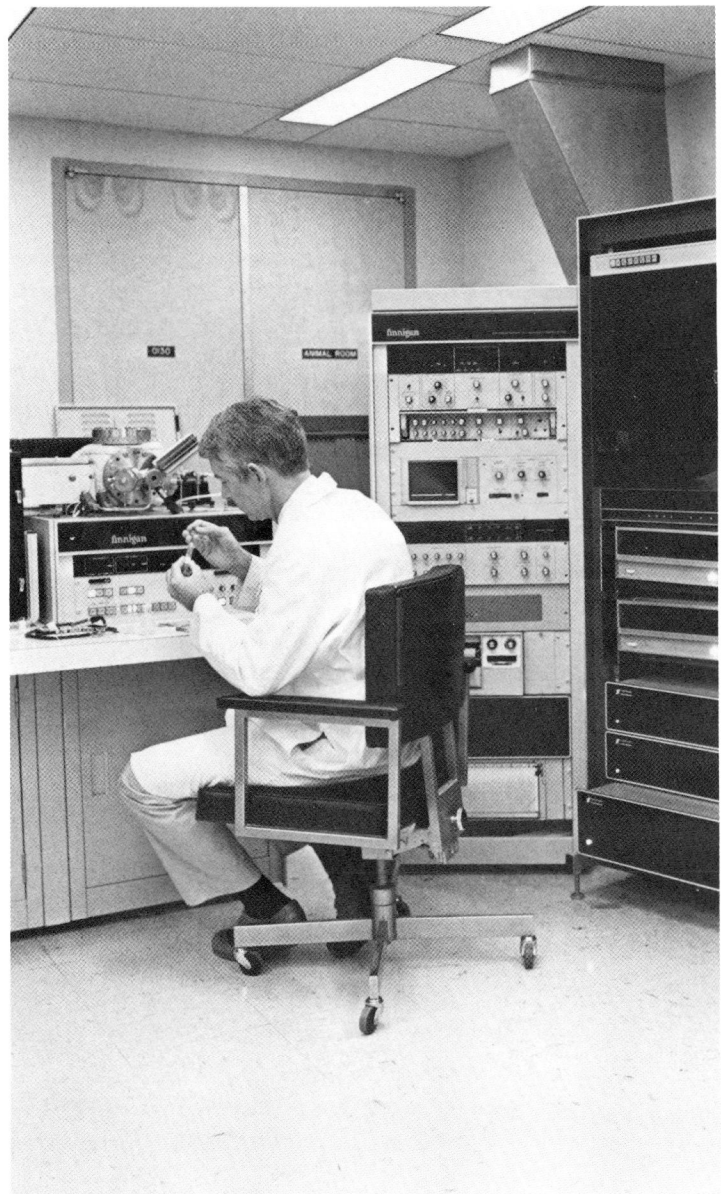

Veterinary research has come a long way since the days of Dr. Townshend and Professor Detmers. Today researchers can rely on dramatically advanced technology in their efforts to protect both animal and human health. (Jeff Bates, OVMA)

It is not recorded, but when OSU approved a 35 percent increase in freshman enrollment in the veterinary college as a response to the post-war boom, someone must have asked the obvious question: "Where will we put them?" Because, in terms of buildings, the College of Veterinary Medicine, one of the largest and most academically progressive in the nation, was still living off the largesse of turn-of-the-century legislatures. Not a single new veterinary structure had gone up since 1910.

It was not for lack of effort. In preceding years, there had been persistent attempts to expand the Veterinary College's physical plant but first the Depression and then World War II intervened. By 1947, the situation was critical and Dean Walter Krill was spelling it out to the OVMA Annual Meeting, including in his remarks some interesting comparisons:

> One of the chief problems preventing the expansion of our college program is the lack of adequate physical plant. When you consider that there had been no building for the College of Veterinary Medicine since 1910, and the only expansion has been largely into makeshift quarters, the necessity becomes quite obvious.... Our buildings ... are inadequate for modern day clinical teaching ... since 1930 there has been talk of new buildings (but) while we have been talking other colleges have been building and expanding their facilities.... Illinois and California are planning to spend from $2,000,000 to $5,000,000 on physical plants for their new colleges. If we are to maintain our position as one of the leading veterinary colleges ... a building program for the college can no longer be delayed.

But delayed it was; the bricks-and-mortar patient would remain on the critical list for several more years. However, the pressure for action was mounting. At its 1952 Annual Meeting, the OVMA reaffirmed its support for Veterinary College construction, responding to a recommendation from President-Elect James T. Burris that the Association "go on record as recognizing the need for a complete new group of buildings for the College of Veterinary Medicine at Ohio State University, if we are to maintain our position and service in this respect to Ohio. Also, that the Association will assist the University in any feasible manner that we can in this connection...."

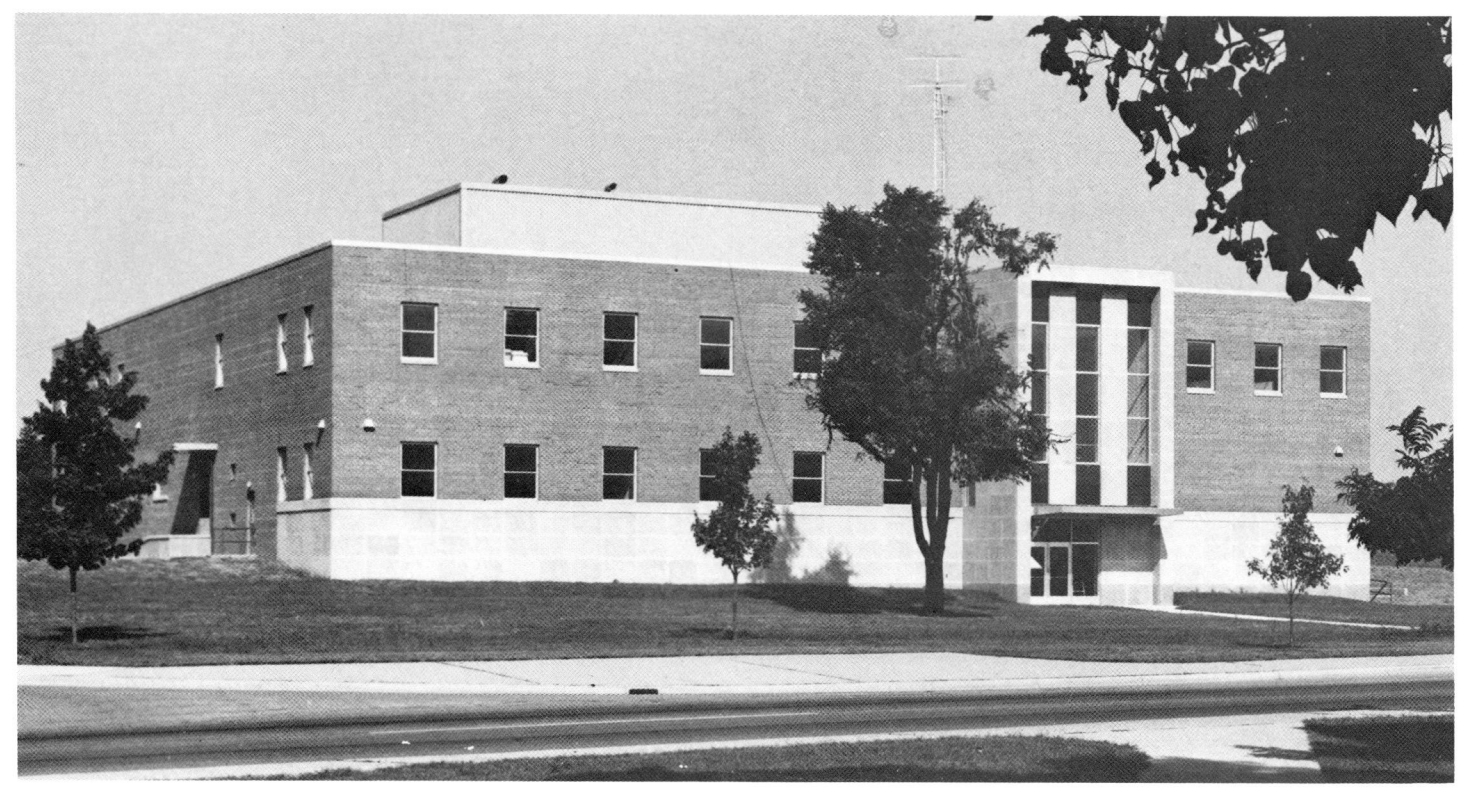

The second new building, the Leonard W. Goss Laboratory, dedicated in 1963. (Department of Photography, Ohio State University)

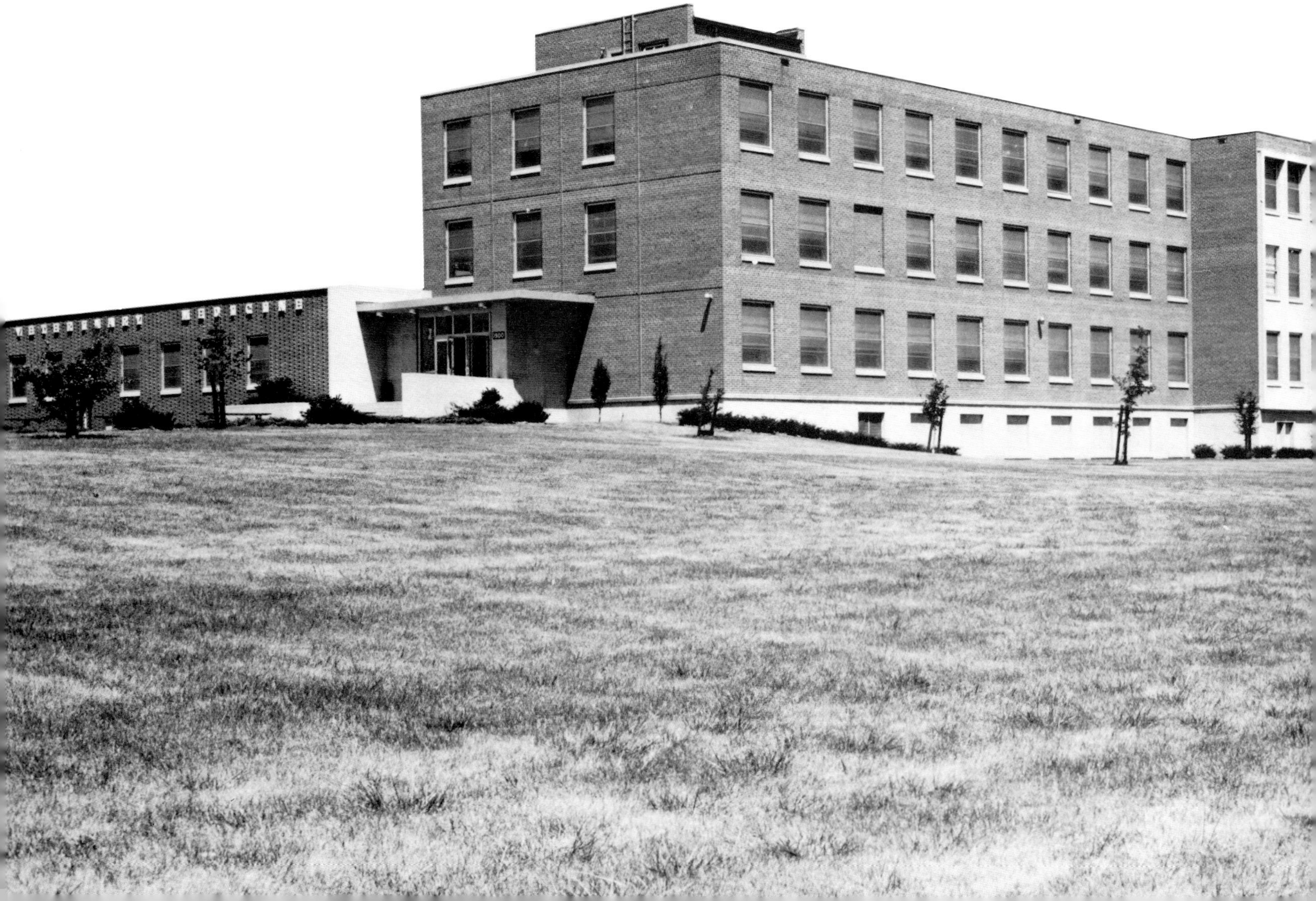

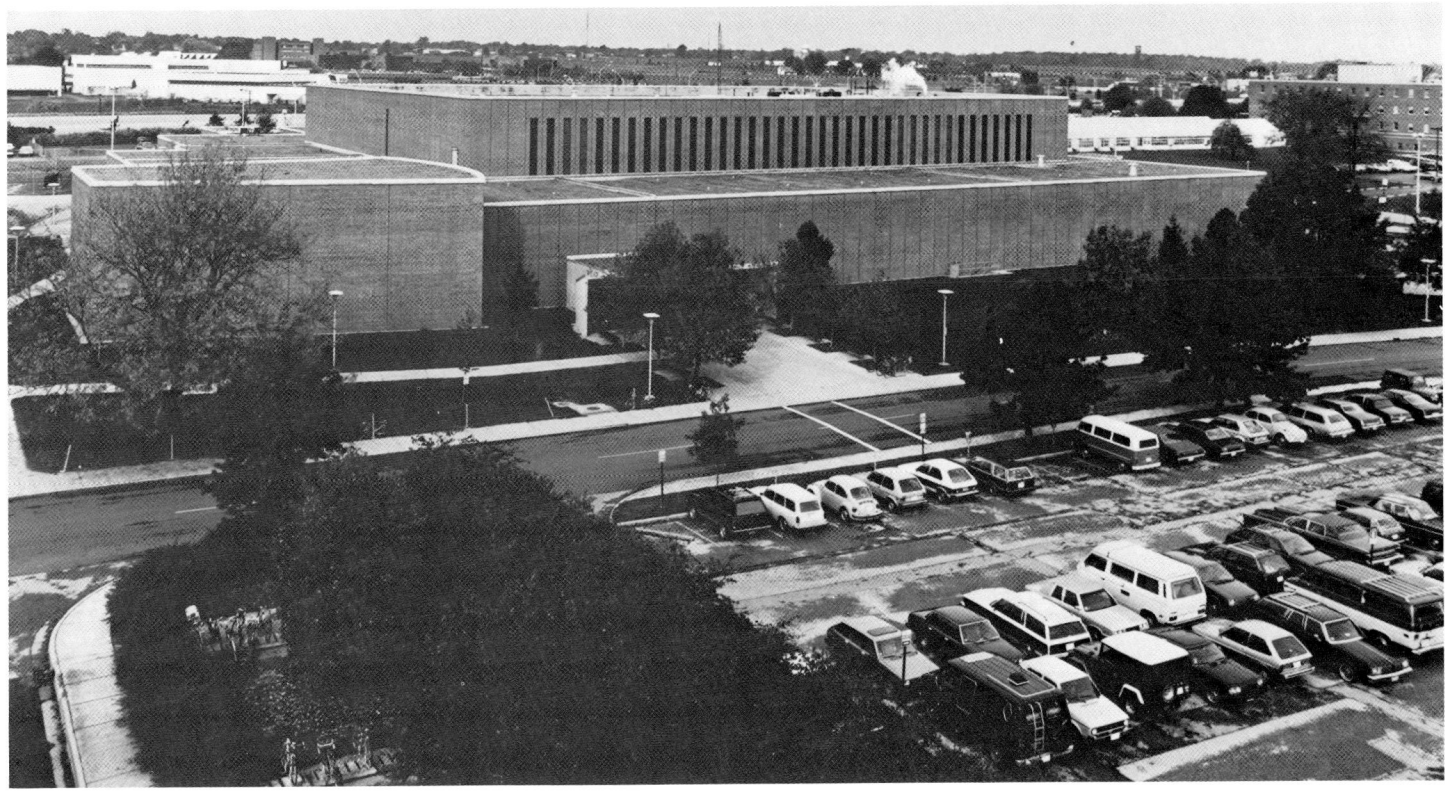

The Veterinary Clinic, dedicated in 1973, was the third phase of College expansion. Still to come is a new Veterinary Sciences facility. (Jeff Bates, OVMA)

The commitment of the OVMA, strong support from state agricultural organizations and the continuing efforts of the Veterinary College itself finally turned the tide. The construction hiatus of nearly 50 years came to an end and the College began to acquire its "new group of buildings."

The first was Sisson Hall, constructed in 1956 at a cost of $2,000,000. Named in honor of Dr. Septimus Sisson, one of the college's early and most distinguished faculty members, it was built to house the basic science departments as well as administrative offices.

Seven years later, the new Leonard W. Goss laboratory opened its doors. The new home of the College's department of veterinary pathology, it was named in honor of the educator who had served as professor and chairman of veterinary pathology from 1920 to 1947.

And, in 1973, the new Veterinary Clinic was dedicated. Built at a cost of $9,000,000 ($5,000,000 in federal funds), the clinic is three times larger than the previous facility and provides an improved teaching environment for veterinary students through advanced equipment and clinical facilities.

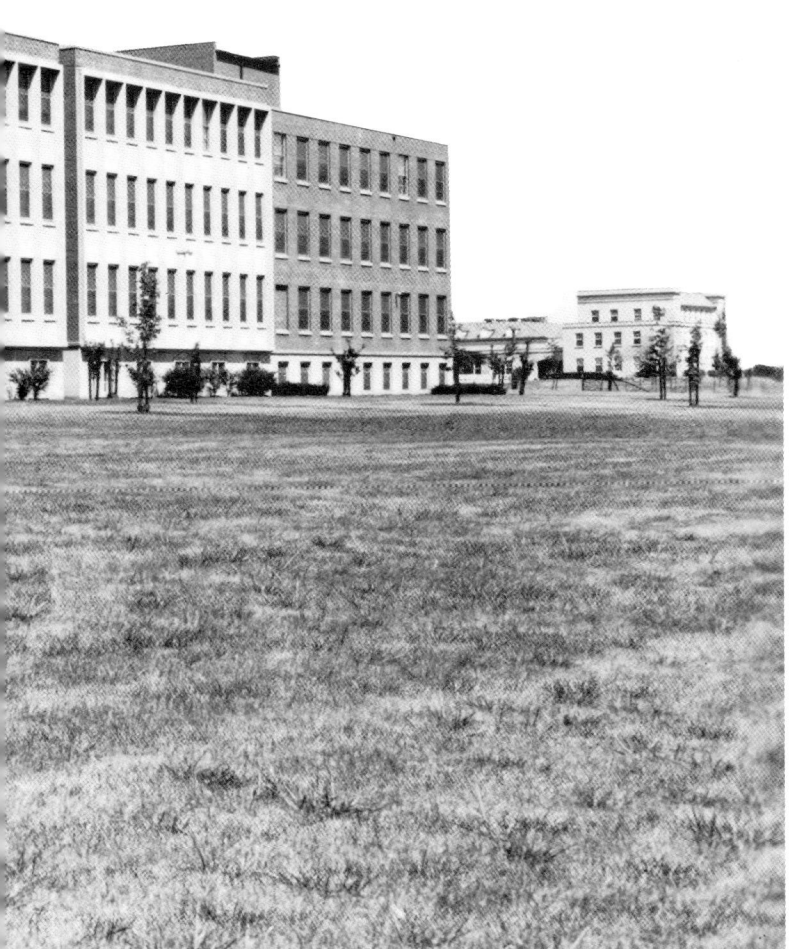

Sisson Hall, constructed in 1956. Named in honor of Dr. Septimus Sisson, it was the Veterinary College's first new building in nearly 50 years. (Photo Archives, Ohio State University)

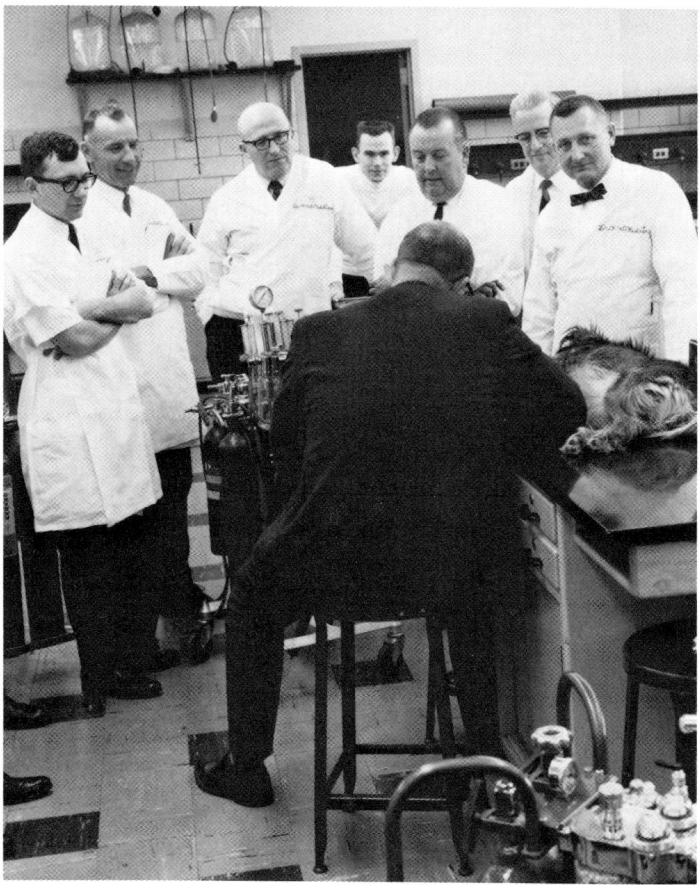

A checkup for the first dog at the Veterinary College to survive open heart surgery. (Photo Archives, Ohio State University)

Today, these three buildings comprise the central campus of the OSU College of Veterinary Medicine. (A fourth structure, a new Veterinary Sciences facility, still awaits financing). They are state-of-the-art facilities, exactly what is required by a College, the third oldest in the nation, which has the largest total enrollment and which has graduated more veterinarians than any other institution.

The OVMA role in promoting Veterinary College expansion is just one example of the cooperative relationship that has prevailed between the College and the Association since the earliest years. OVMA help in sponsoring OSU's annual Veterinary Conferences is another; this program began in 1927 and continued until 1950 when, with continued Association support, it was replaced by intensified short courses covering subject matter in greater depth.

The Association also has provided financial support for the Ohio State Fair Live Surgery Exhibit, a continuing project of the OSU Student Chapter of the AVMA. And there has been continued emphasis on the OVMA Preceptorship, initiated in 1968. This program, an adaptation of an earlier intern program developed by practicing veterinarians (notably Drs. Claude H. Case and John F. Planz, partners in the Akron Veterinary Hospital) is designed to link veterinary students with practitioners to provide practical training not entirely available in colleges. Since the

The Ohio State Fair Live Surgery Exhibit, a continuing project of the OSU Student Chapter of the AVMA, receives financial support from the OVMA. (OVMA files)

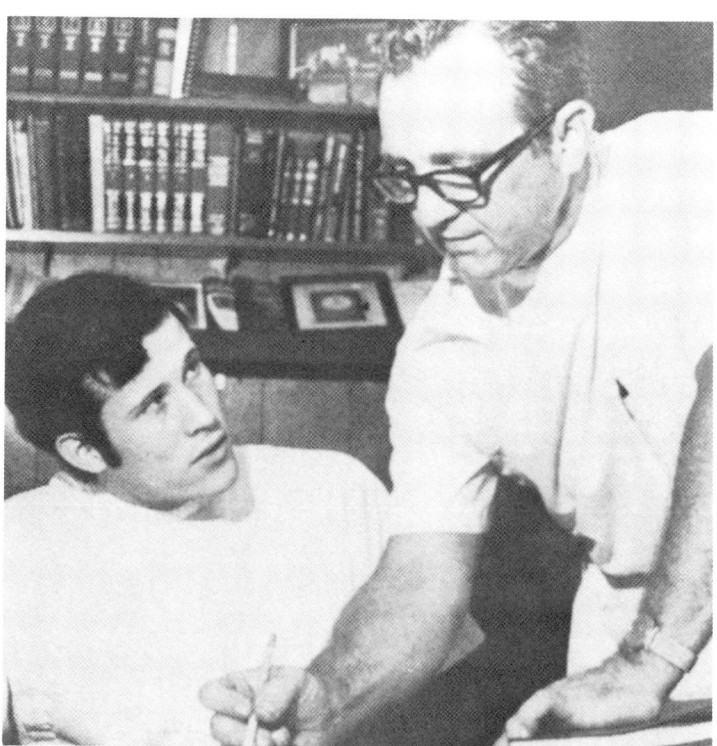

In 1968, the OVMA launched a Preceptorship Program to link veterinary students with established practitioners. In this 1969 photo, Dr. J. Bruce Wenger shares his skills and knowledge with Preceptor Robert Brown. (OVMA files)

program began, 296 students have worked in a preceptorship relationship with 156 participating veterinarians.

Veterinary Research at OSU

Since the days when Dr. Norton Townshend cited the importance of "carefully and skillfully conducted" investigations of animal disease and Professor H. J. Detmers undertook "experiments for the purpose of ascertaining the true cause or causes of some infectious diseases," research has been an integral part of veterinary medicine at OSU.

In the first decades, the strongest emphasis was on large animal research, an obvious result of the importance of the horse and the devastating impact of livestock diseases such as hog cholera, bovine tuberculosis, and brucellosis. But as veterinary medicine broadened its scope, the OSU Veterinary College (and other veterinary schools) also greatly expanded their research programs. With the rapid growth of small animal practice, research in this area took on increased importance and the same period saw the formation of a crucial research alliance between human and animal medicine.

The range of veterinary research and its importance to both animal and human health were effectively summed up on May 13, 1983, by Dr. W. Ann Reynolds, former OSU provost and now chancellor of The California State University. In a presentation for Phi Zeta Research Day at the OSU

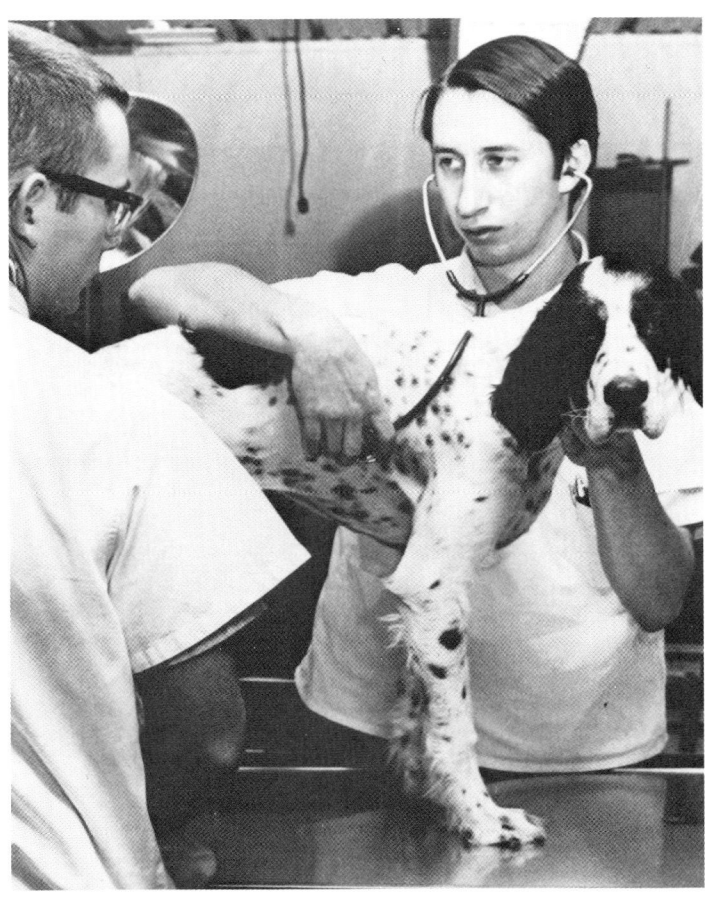

A continuing education short course at the Veterinary College, 1968. Over the years, continuing education programs at OSU have had the strong support of the OVMA. (Photo Archives, Ohio State University)

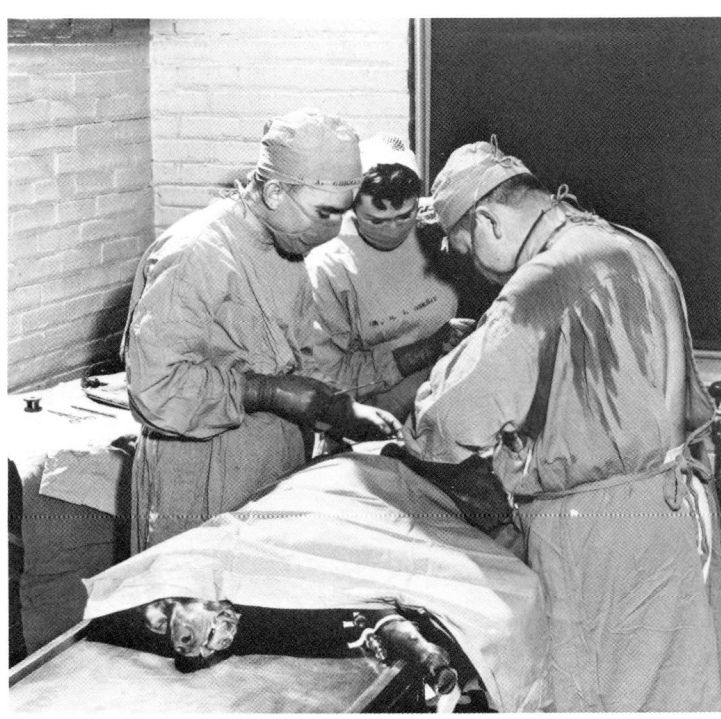

A 1955 operation to fit a dog with the Gorman hip replacement prosthesis. Dr. Gorman's artificial hip was hailed as a major advance in orthopedics. (Photo Archives, Ohio State University)

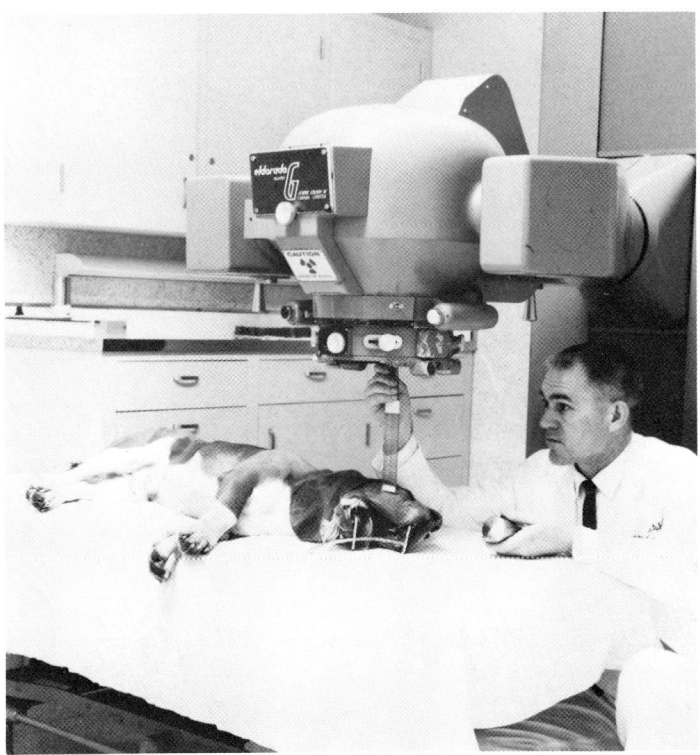

Cobalt therapy for a dog at the OSU Veterinary College, 1963. (Photo Archives, Ohio State University)

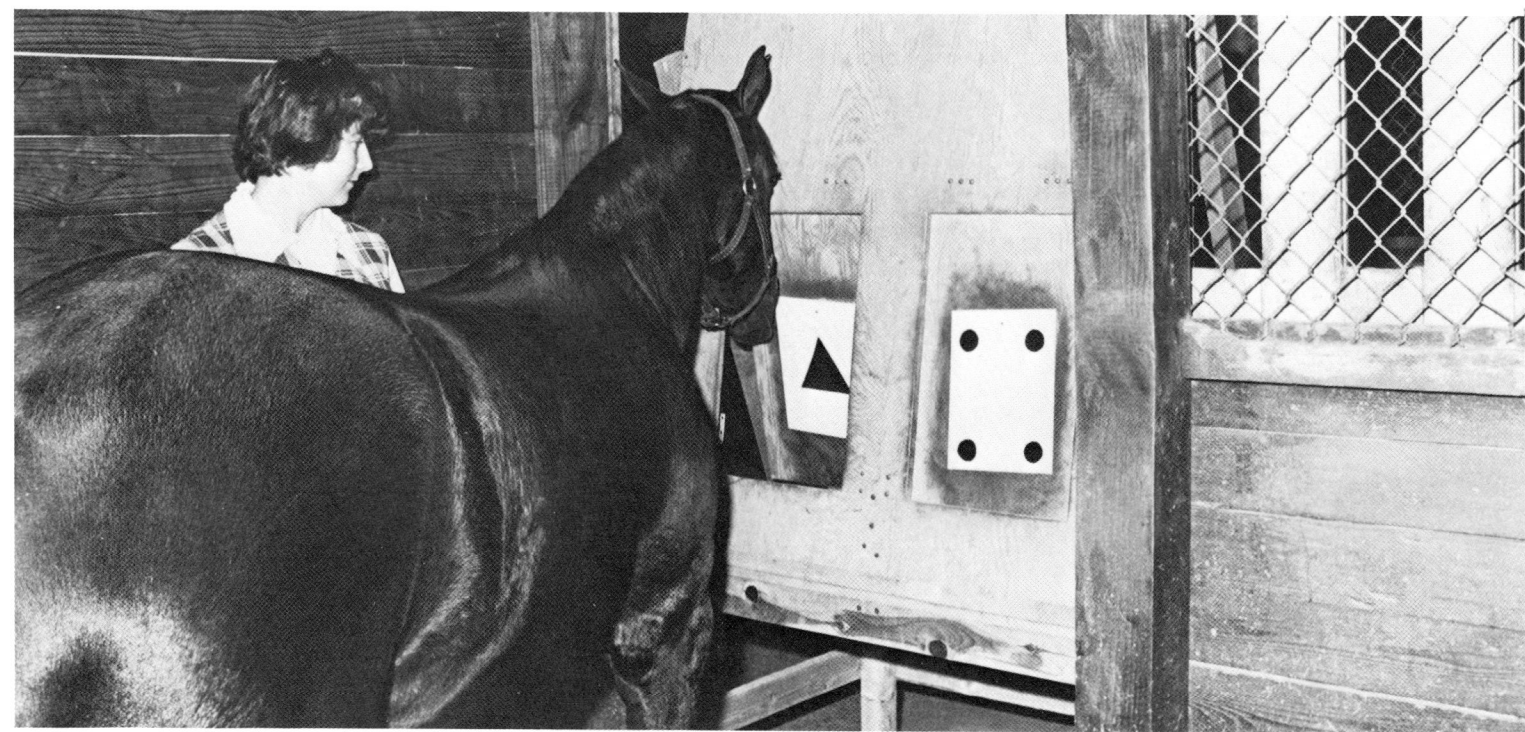

Animal intelligence also is a field for veterinary research. Here, Dr. Victoria Voith tests a horse's intelligence by seeing if it can differentiate between geometric symbols. (Photo Archives, Ohio State University)

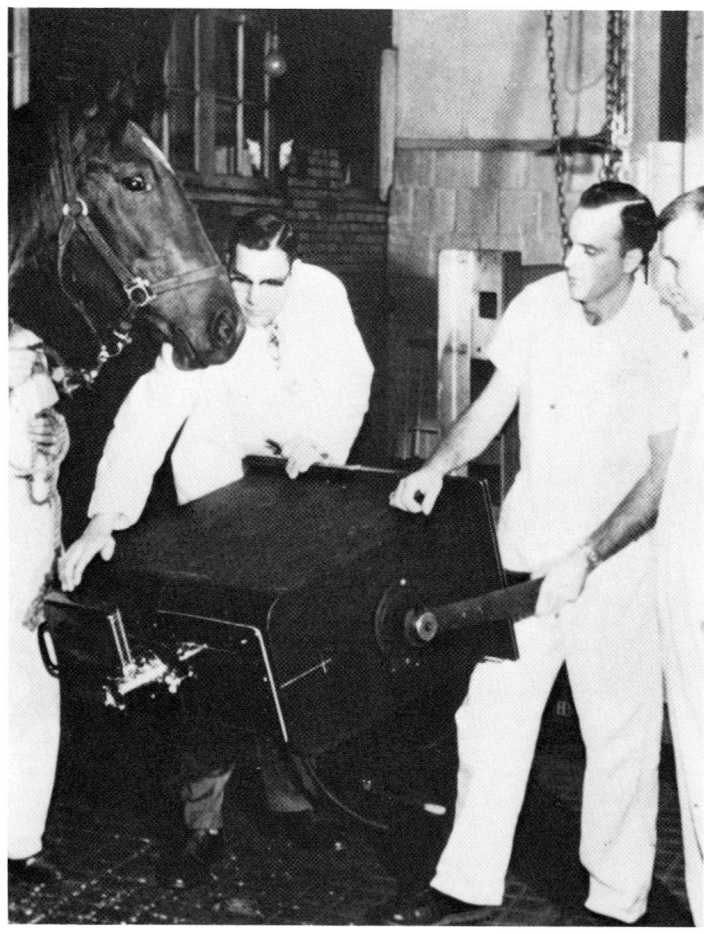

Veterinary students learn the fine art of handling a portable X-Ray machine. (Photo Archives, Ohio State University)

Veterinary College, she cited an impressive list of veterinary "firsts":

> ... the pinning techniques used in fracture reduction, the first hip replacement prosthesis, the first hypodermic syringe, the first successful hookworm therapy, artificial insemination, the first electrocardiogram, cardiac catheterization, and the first spinal anesthesia, all were developed in veterinary rather than human medical research. Even today, in chemotherapy, immunology and many other important areas, experimental medicine is still largely animal medicine. The use of animal models for the study of human diseases is an important and growing area of veterinary research.... Well over 250 animal models for human diseases have been identified and many more probably await discovery.

The hip replacement prosthesis noted by Dr. Reynolds was an OSU achievement; working at the Veterinary College, Air Force Colonel and veterinarian Dr. Harry Gorman developed an artifical hip for dogs far superior to existing designs. Hailed by Columbus orthopedic surgeon Dr. Judson W. Wilson as "one of the greatest advancements in orthopedics in the last 100 years," the Gorman hip joint was successfully adapted with modifications for use in human prothesis.

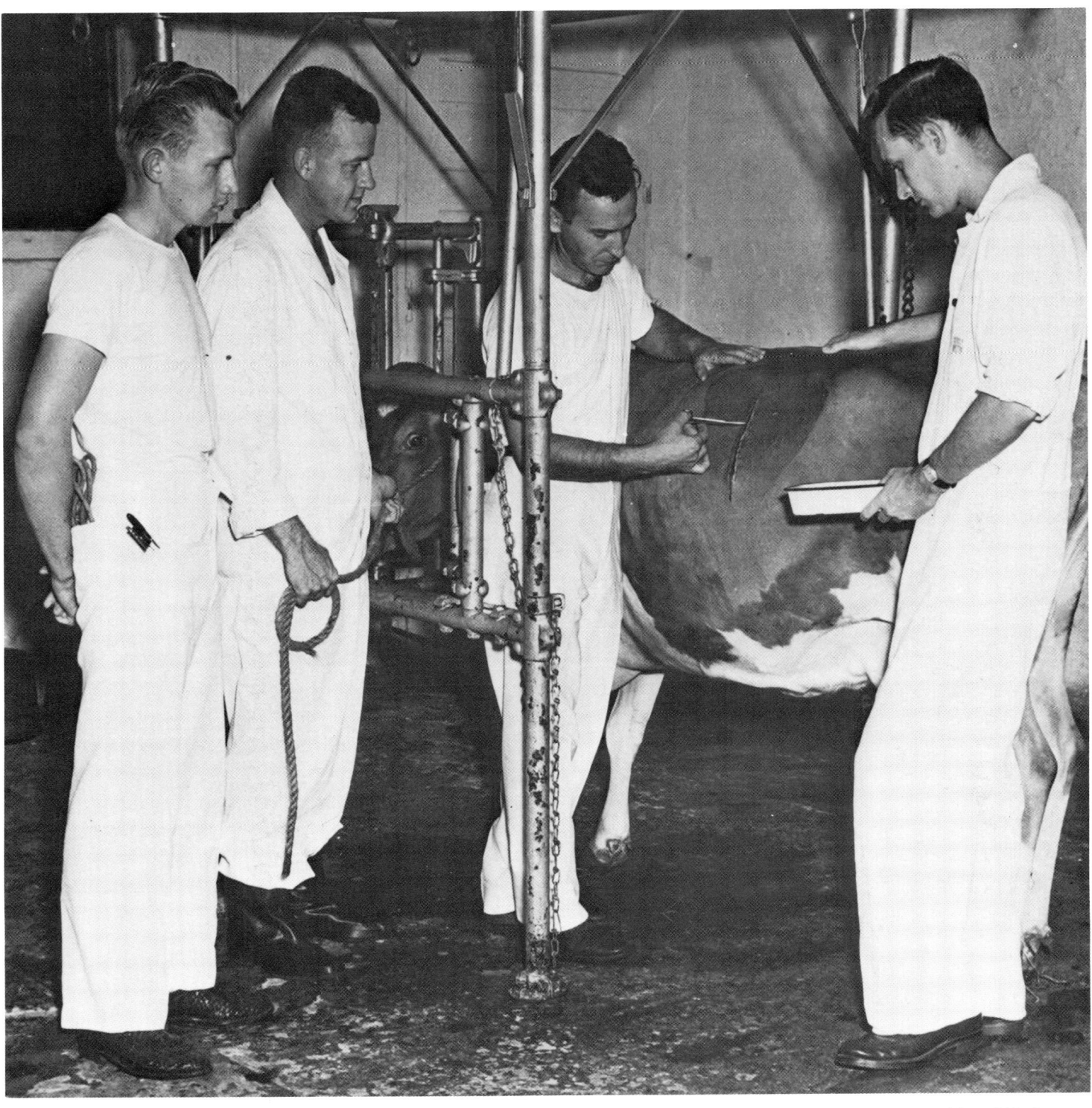
Veterinary students skillfully incise a cow in a 1950 demonstration at the Ohio State Fair. The cow doesn't seem to mind. (Photo Archives, Ohio State University)

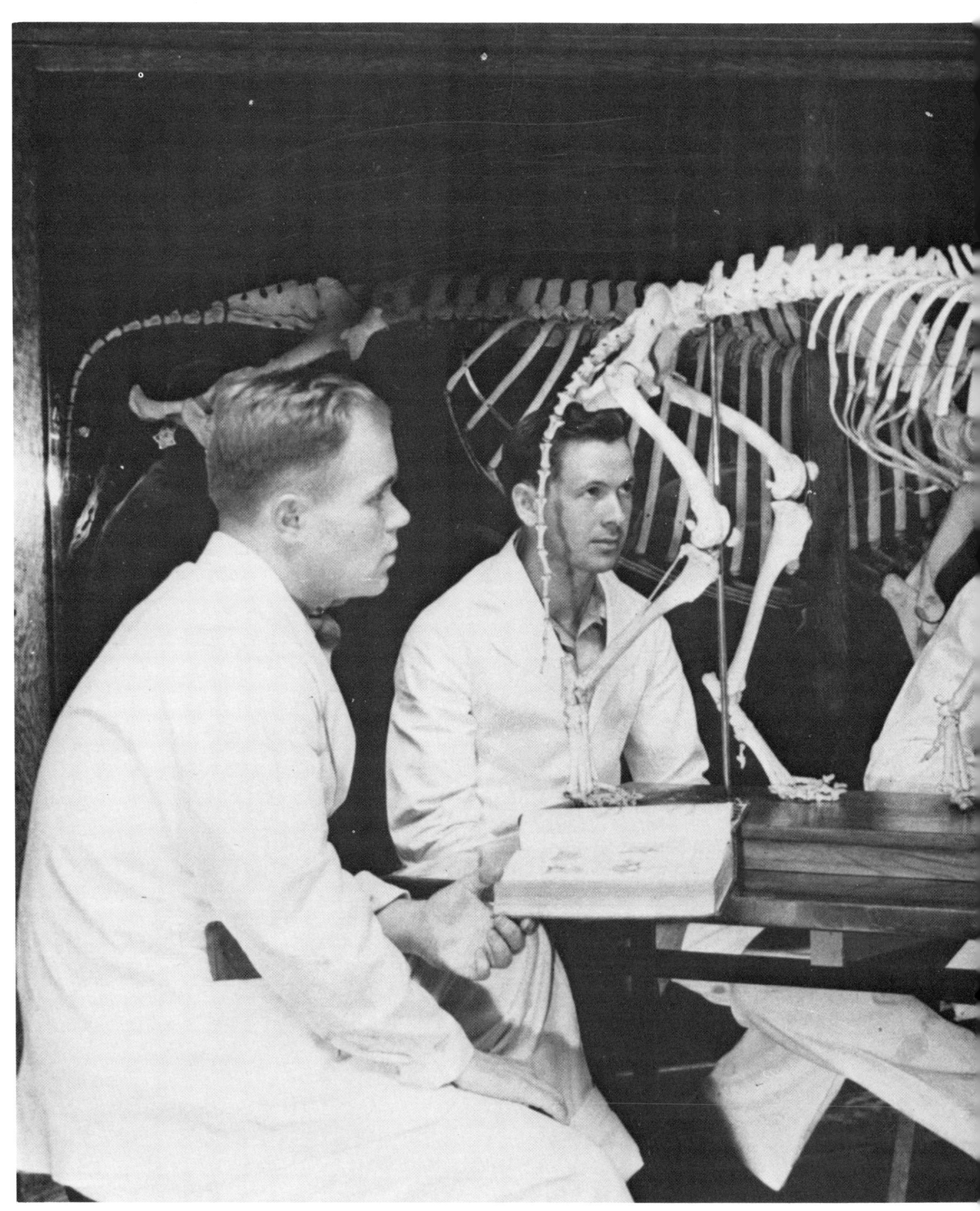

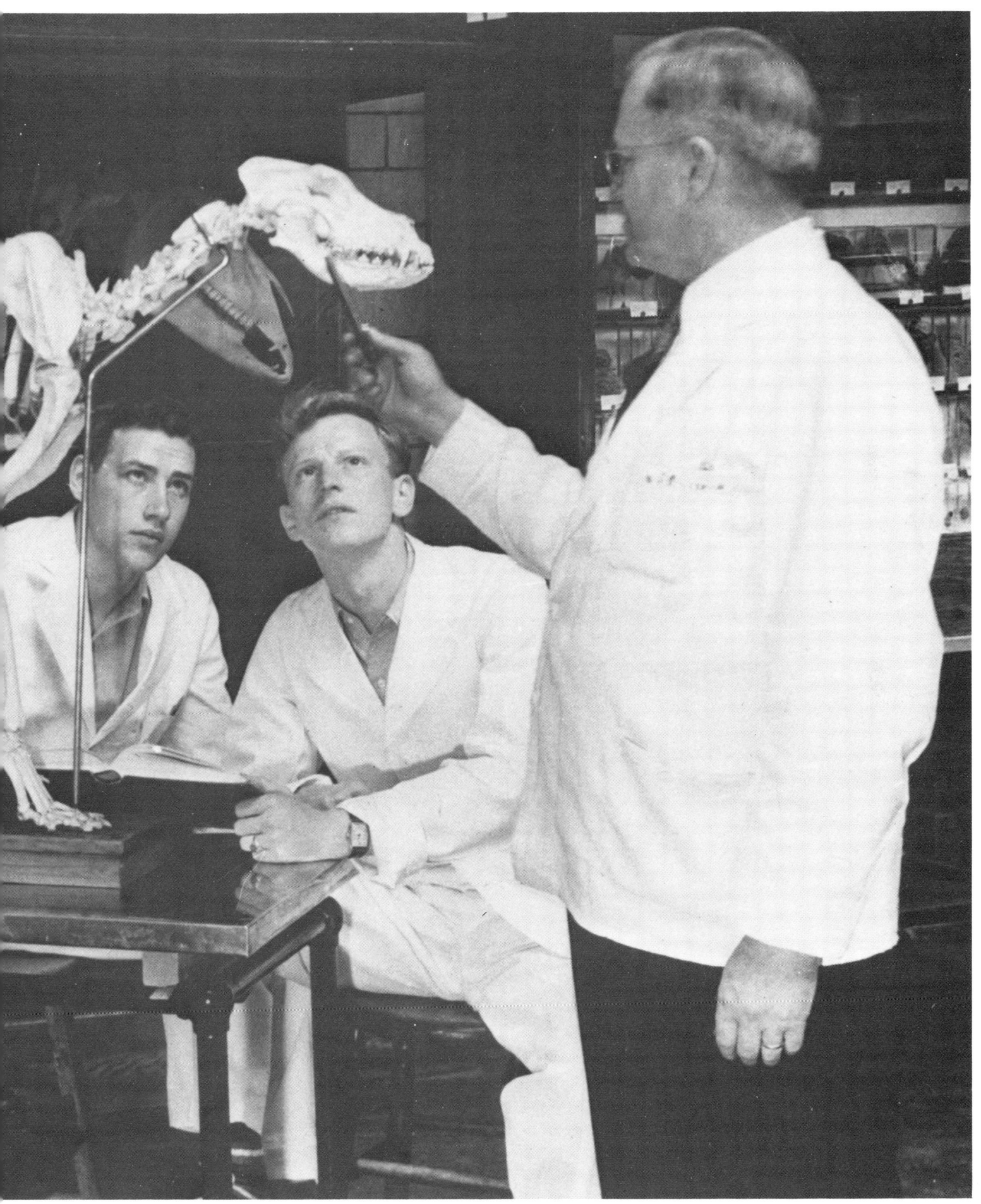
Explaining some of the finer points of animal anatomy during a 1948 class session. (Photo Archives, Ohio State University)

A CENTURY OF CARING

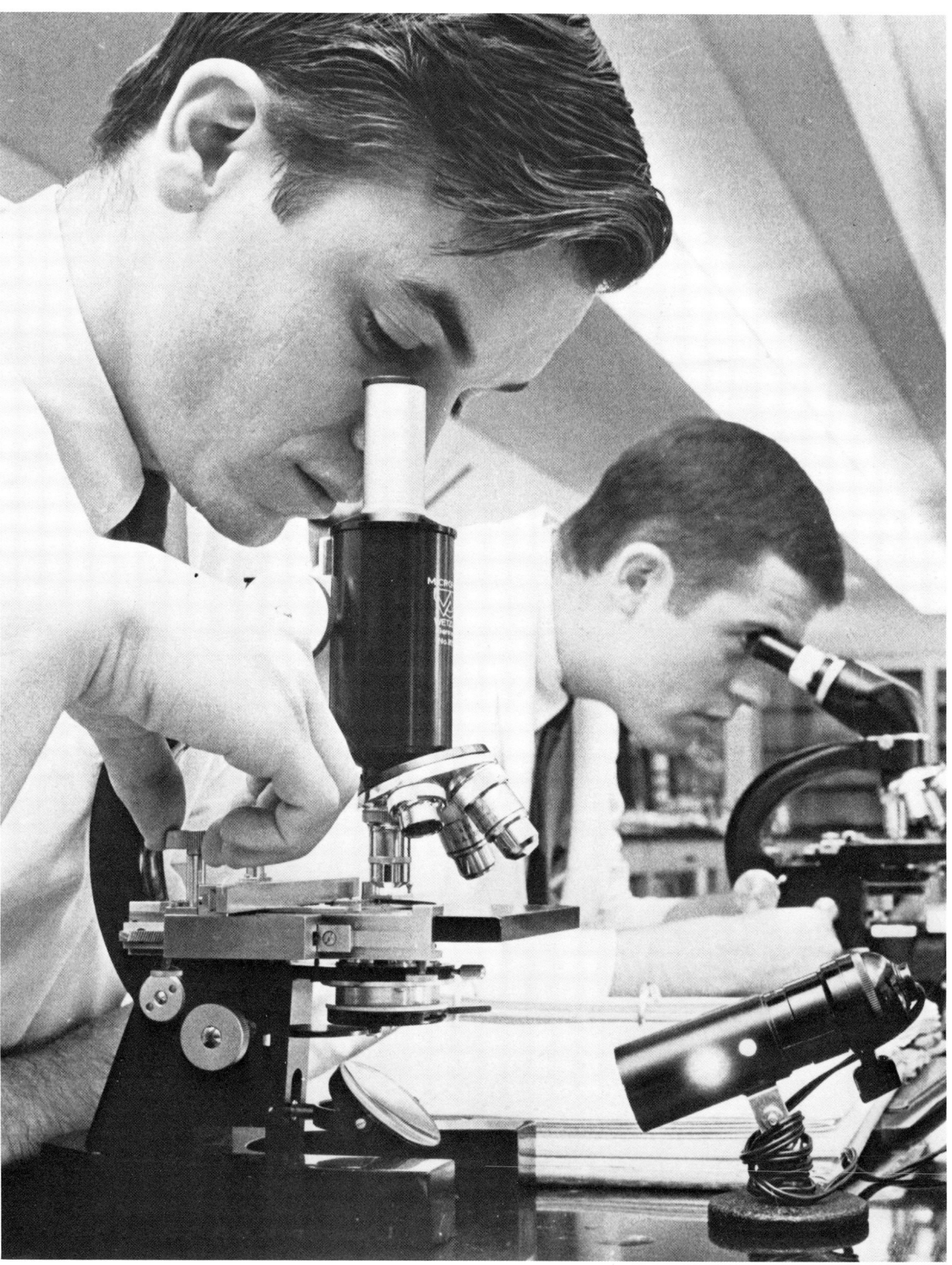

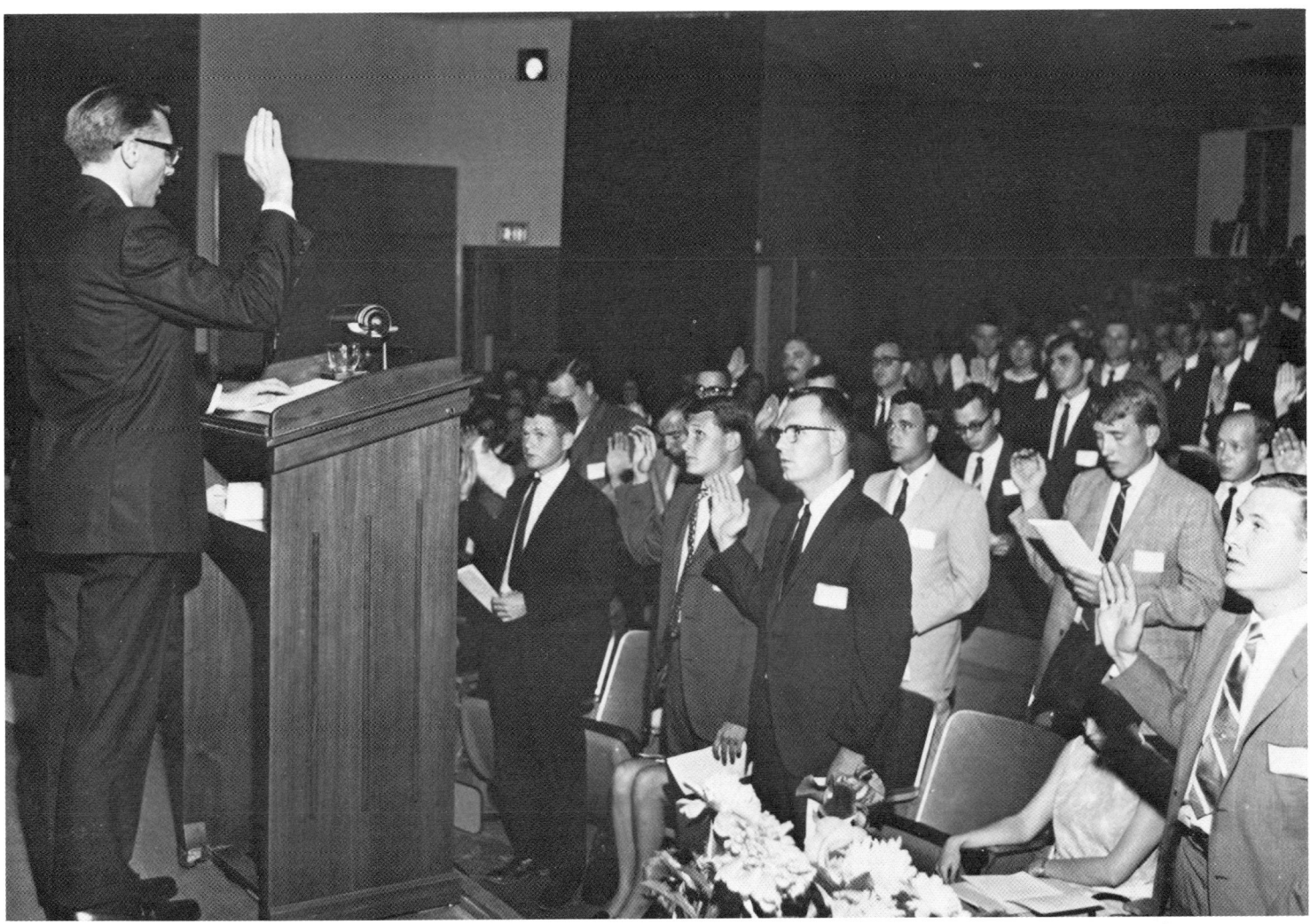

The closing of one chapter, the beginning of another. Members of the Class of 1968 take the Veterinarians' Oath. (Photo Archives, Ohio State University)

Other OSU Veterinary College research achievements have included pioneering work in the development of an effective vaccine against feline leukemia and major studies of the canine distemper virus. The Veterinary College also has made extensive studies of heart valve irregularities in horses, compiling data of great value to researchers in the field of human heart disease.

Always important, veterinary medical research at OSU began a period of particularly dramatic growth in the late 1960s. This rapid expansion, reflected in the annual reports of the OSU Research Foundation, has been marked by an almost ten-fold increase in veterinary research expenditures.

In 1968, the Veterinary College was engaged in a total of 18 research projects, with expenditures totalling $240,000. By 1973, the number of projects had almost doubled (35) and research spending was close

Future veterinarians hit the microscopes in 1976. (Photo Archives, Ohio State University)

to $1,000,000. Five years later, in 1978, there were 57 projects with spending of $1,400,000. And in 1982, 76 projects were underway at the College, with research expenditures of over $2,000,000.

Current veterinary research at OSU is characterized by the wide variety of research projects. Large animal studies are still important, indicative of the continuing needs of the livestock industry, but these efforts are matched by extensive small animal research, in part the result of the steady expansion of small animal practice. There is also increased emphasis on equine research, a response to the comeback of the horse. And of great significance in recent years has been veterinary medicine's growing participation in the field of cancer research. At OSU, several projects have involved cooperative efforts between the Veterinary College, the Medical School and the Cancer Research Center, further confirmation of the important partnership that now links animal and human medical research.

A CENTURY OF CARING

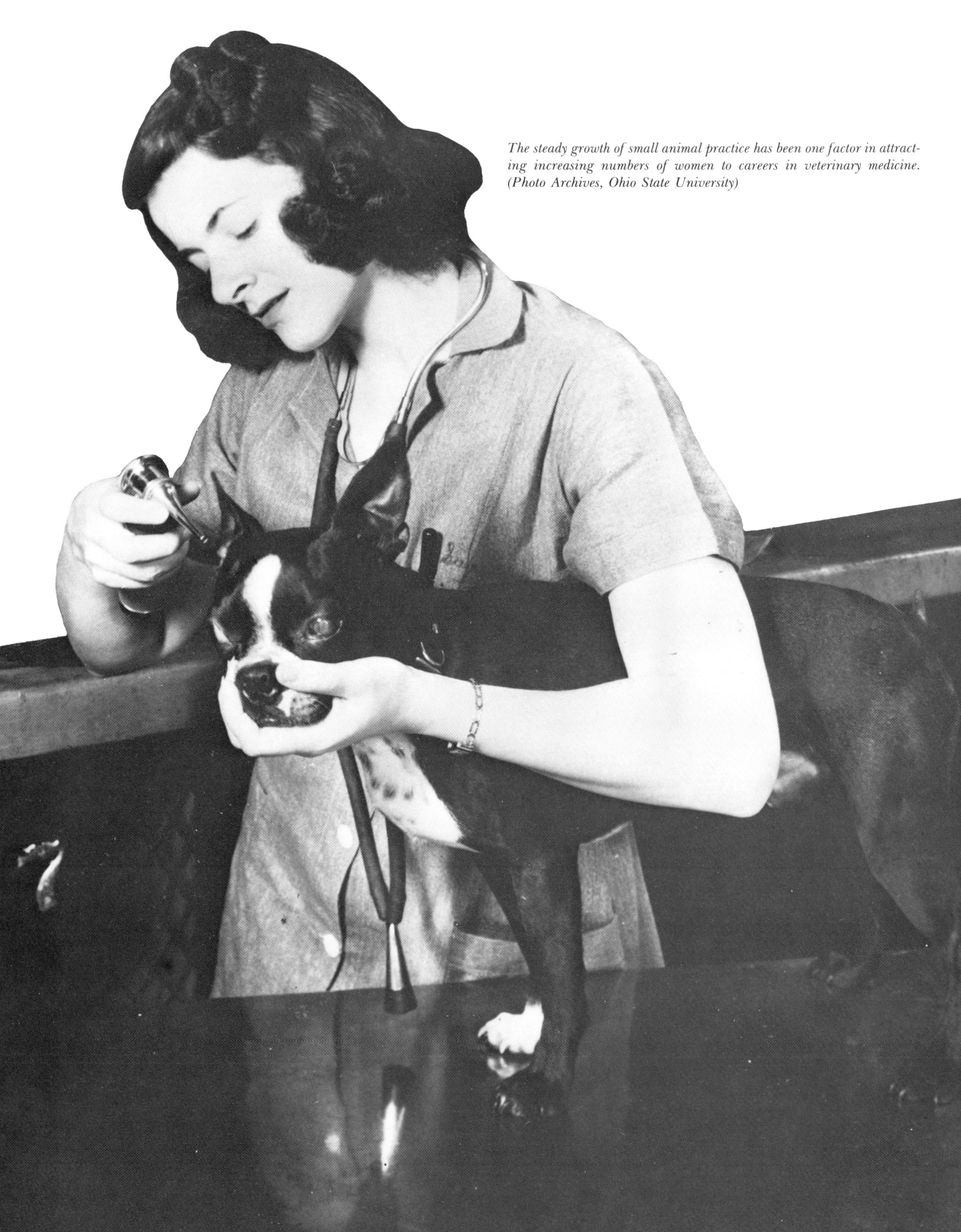

The steady growth of small animal practice has been one factor in attracting increasing numbers of women to careers in veterinary medicine. (Photo Archives, Ohio State University)

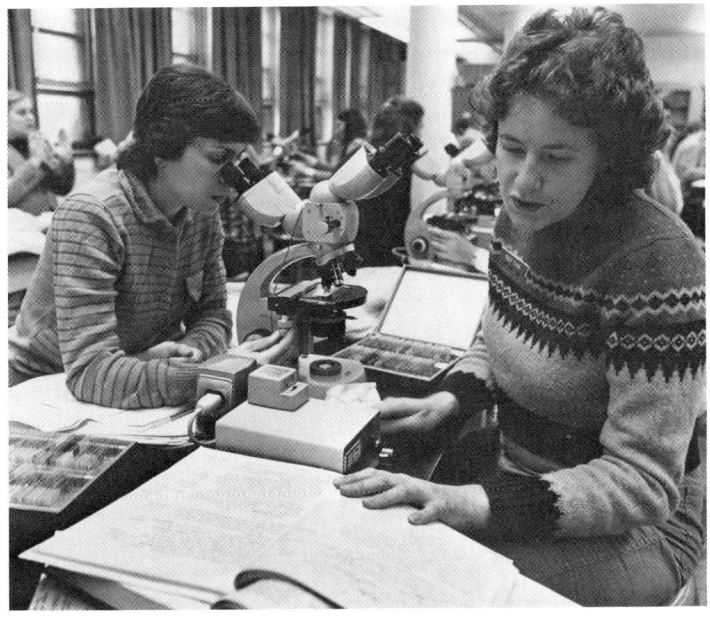
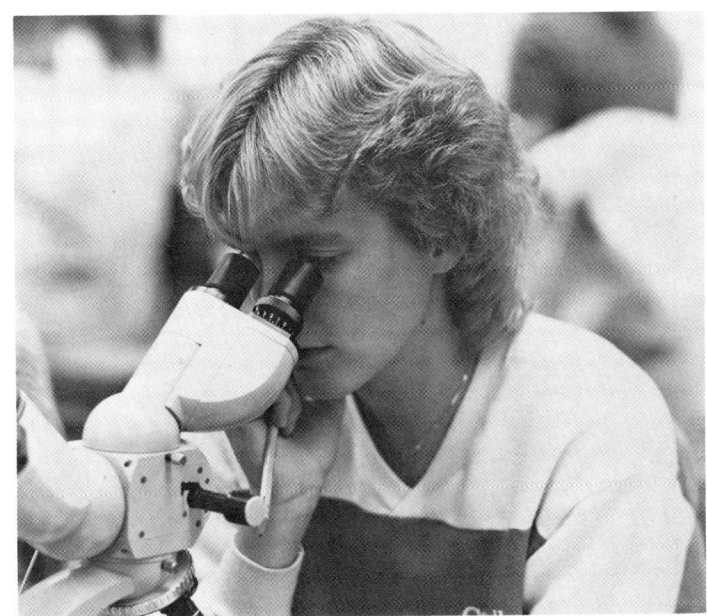

Not For Men Only

For most of its history, veterinary medicine remained a distinctly masculine discipline. Prevailing opinion on the "proper" role of women and the rigors of veterinary practice combined to stamp the profession "For Men Only" and this injunction presented a formidable obstacle to women seeking to enter the field.

In the early years a few did persist and prevail; in 1903, Mignon Nicholson became the first American woman veterinarian upon her graduation from McKillip Veterinary College in Chicago, and seven years later, in 1910, Florence Kimball graduated from the Veterinary College of Cornell University. But these were exceptions to the rule. For decades to come, men continued to almost completely dominate the profession, still secure in their belief that women not only did not belong in veterinary medicine but simply could not do the work.

In 1934, there still were only 16 women veterinarians in the United States. And almost 30 years later, in 1963, out of a record U.S. veterinary college enrollment of 3,727, only 190 were women.

The OSU Veterinary College graduated its first woman, Ida Mae Dodge, in June, 1936. From then on, the College had one woman graduate a year through 1959, with the exception of 1949 when four women graduated. In the 1960s, there was a slight increase in the number of women graduates; throughout the decade the College averaged three women per graduating class. Still, 85 years after its founding, the Veterinary College remained very much a man's world.

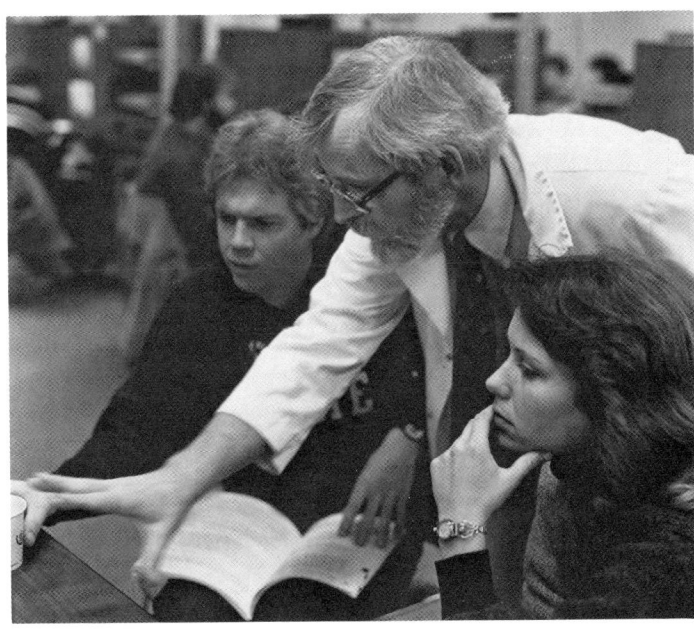

Veterinary education is now a woman's as well as a man's world. Over the past decade, the enrollment of women students in the OSU Veterinary College has risen sharply and today it equals and sometimes exceeds male enrollment. (Jeff Bates, OVMA)

But times were changing. The growth of small animal practice and veterinary research opened new avenues of opportunity for women, and in the large animal field, new handling techniques, including tranquilizers and mechanical hoisting devices, were eliminating sheer physical strength as a prerequisite for veterinary practice. There also were changes in public attitudes, a significant one being cited in a 1976 study, "Women in Veterinary Medicine," compiled for the Department of Health, Education and Welfare. The study observed that:

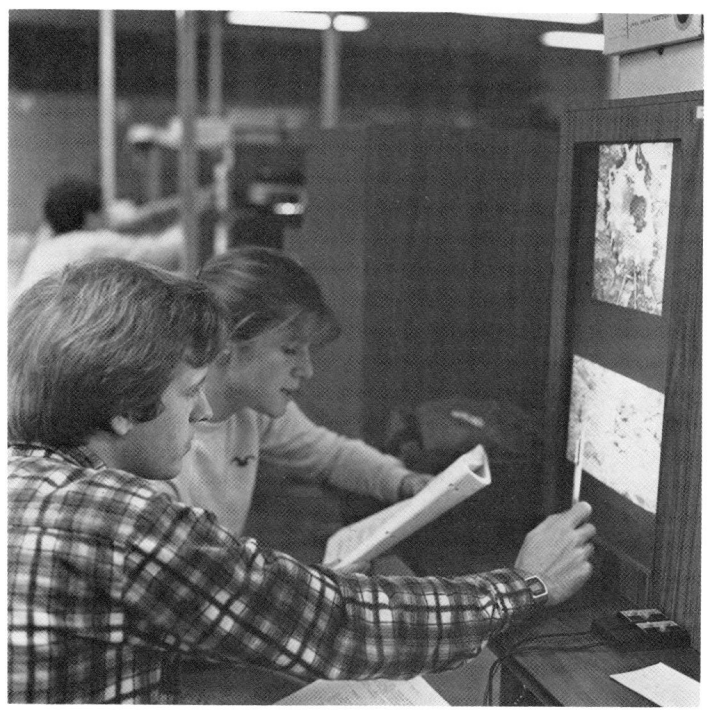

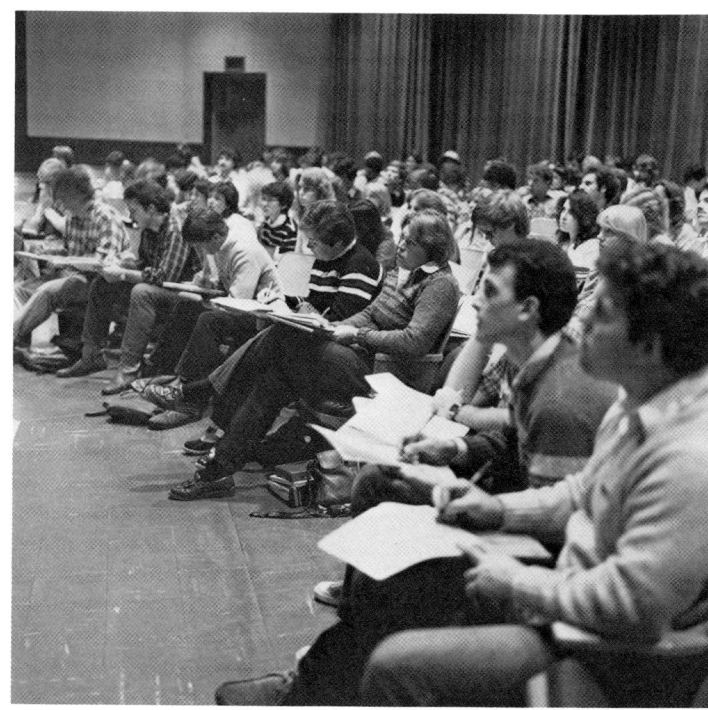

Lectures, individual study and faculty-student interaction are the key elements of veterinary education at OSU, which boasts one of the nation's finest veterinary colleges. (Jeff Bates, OVMA)

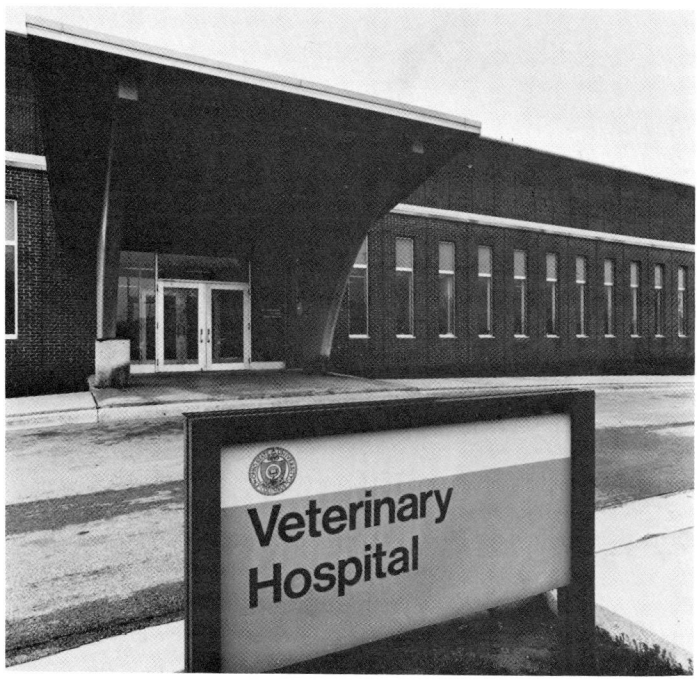

. . . current romantic notions about working with animals have lessened the extreme masculine image of the (veterinary) profession. This allows a woman to do the work without risking total loss of her femininity in the eyes of other people.

The same study also noted that "societal ideas about work have changed and doing physical, outdoor work is seen as less demeaning than it once was."

These factors, together with the growing self-awareness of women and their determination to seek career opportunities in previously male-oriented professions, produced some dramatic changes at the veterinary colleges in a relatively short time. In 1973, for example, the OSU Veterinary College had eight women graduates, a not-very-sizable increase over previous years. But in 1978, the College graduated 38 women, an almost five-fold increase over a six-year period, and in 1980, the number climbed to 54. Fifty-five women graduated from the Veterinary College in 1982 and 61 in 1983.

Paralleling this has been an equally impressive redress in the balance between male and female veterinary students. In enrollment, women have moved into a position of parity; in fact, for the past two years, the OSU Veterinary College has had more women than men in its freshman classes.

The influx of women into the veterinary profession also is reflected in the membership rolls of the OVMA. The Association did not gain its first woman member until 1946, when it admitted Dr. Robertta Laughlin Fitts, a graduate of Ontario Veterinary College. But since then, there has been a steady increase in the number of female members and today the OVMA carries on its rolls over 80 women veterinarians.

"For Men Only" is a thing of the past.

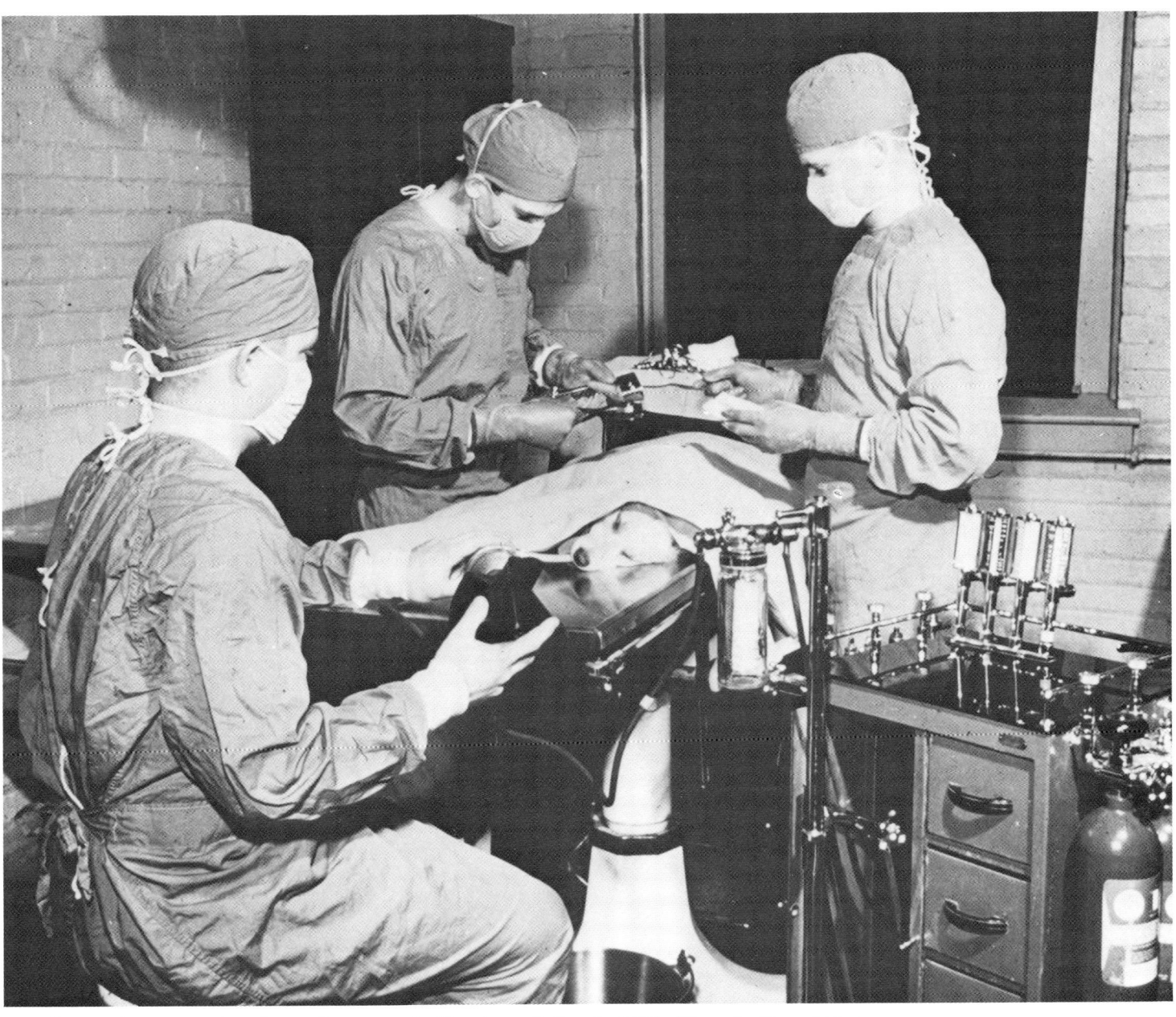
An ailing canine gets another chance. Surgery at the Veterinary College in 1959. (Photo Archives, Ohio State University)

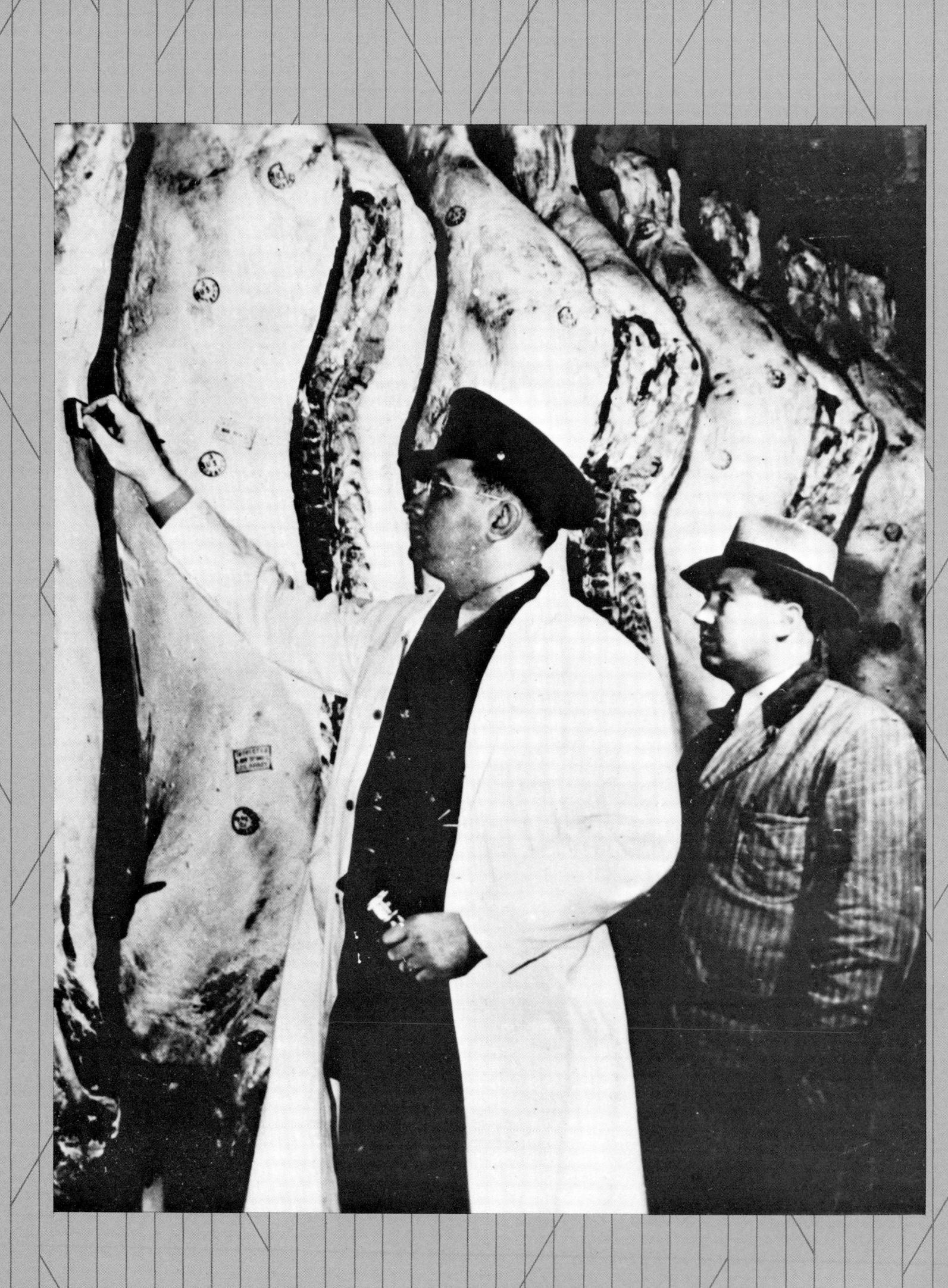

CHAPTER VIII

VETERINARY MEDICINE: THE MILITARY CONNECTION

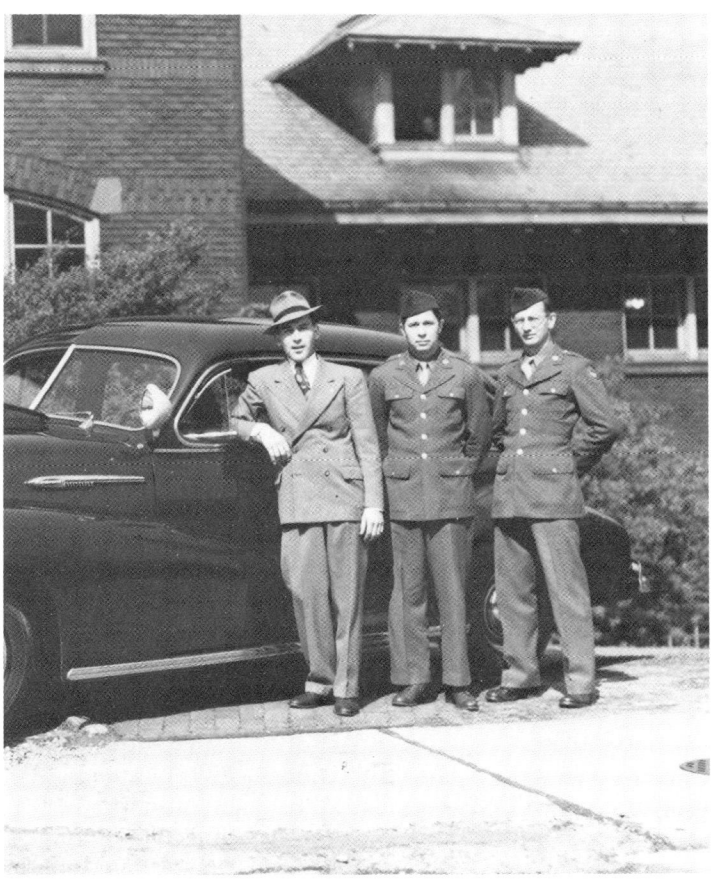

OSU veterinary students in uniform during World War II. When the Army Student Training Program ended in 1944, a number of students suspended their education and enlisted in the Armed Forces, choosing to serve even though they were assured freedom from induction until after graduation. (Photo Archives, Ohio State University)

One of the most important duties of military veterinarians in World War II was food inspection and supervision. Their success in preventing outbreaks of food poisoning greatly enhanced the standing of both the Army Veterinary Corps and the entire profession. (Photo Archives, Ohio State University)

It is accurate to say that through the 1800s, the relationship between professional veterinary medicine and the nation's military establishment was practically nonexistent.

There was, of course, no veterinary service during the Revolutionary War; the rebelling colonies, lagging far behind Europe, had no trained veterinarians. But even when the profession began to take shape in the mid-1800s, the military still ignored its pressing need for a veterinary corps and continued to rely largely on farriers and other untrained personnel for animal care. The Civil War, a costly victory and loss for North and South respectively, was a disaster for the animals involved; only a handful of professional veterinarians served in the military forces (in lower-echelon ranks) and the animal losses from disease and mishandling were staggering.

In the Spanish-American War much the same situation prevailed and although the war's tainted food scandal did focus attention on the need for veterinary inspection of perishable foods, little else was learned from the conflict. The broader importance of veterinary service continued to go unrecognized by military authorities for another two decades.

It was not until the eve of U.S. involvement in World War I that veterinary medicine achieved real status in the military. The occasion was noted at the OVMA's 1917 Annual Meeting in a Progress and Education Committee report that also included a sharp comment about the preceding years:

> Until June 3 of last year, the status of the veterinary service of the United States Army might well be characterized as a disgrace to a civilized nation . . . and a gross injustice to the veterinary profession. The Army Reorganization Act, now officially known as the National Defense Act, went into effect on July 1, 1916. It provides for a Veterinary Corps as a part . . . of the Army . . . veterinarians will have rank, pay and allowances ranging from second lieutenant to major inclusive. . . . It is evidently a source of intense gratification to our profession to have gained this recognition after a long and often discouraging struggle.

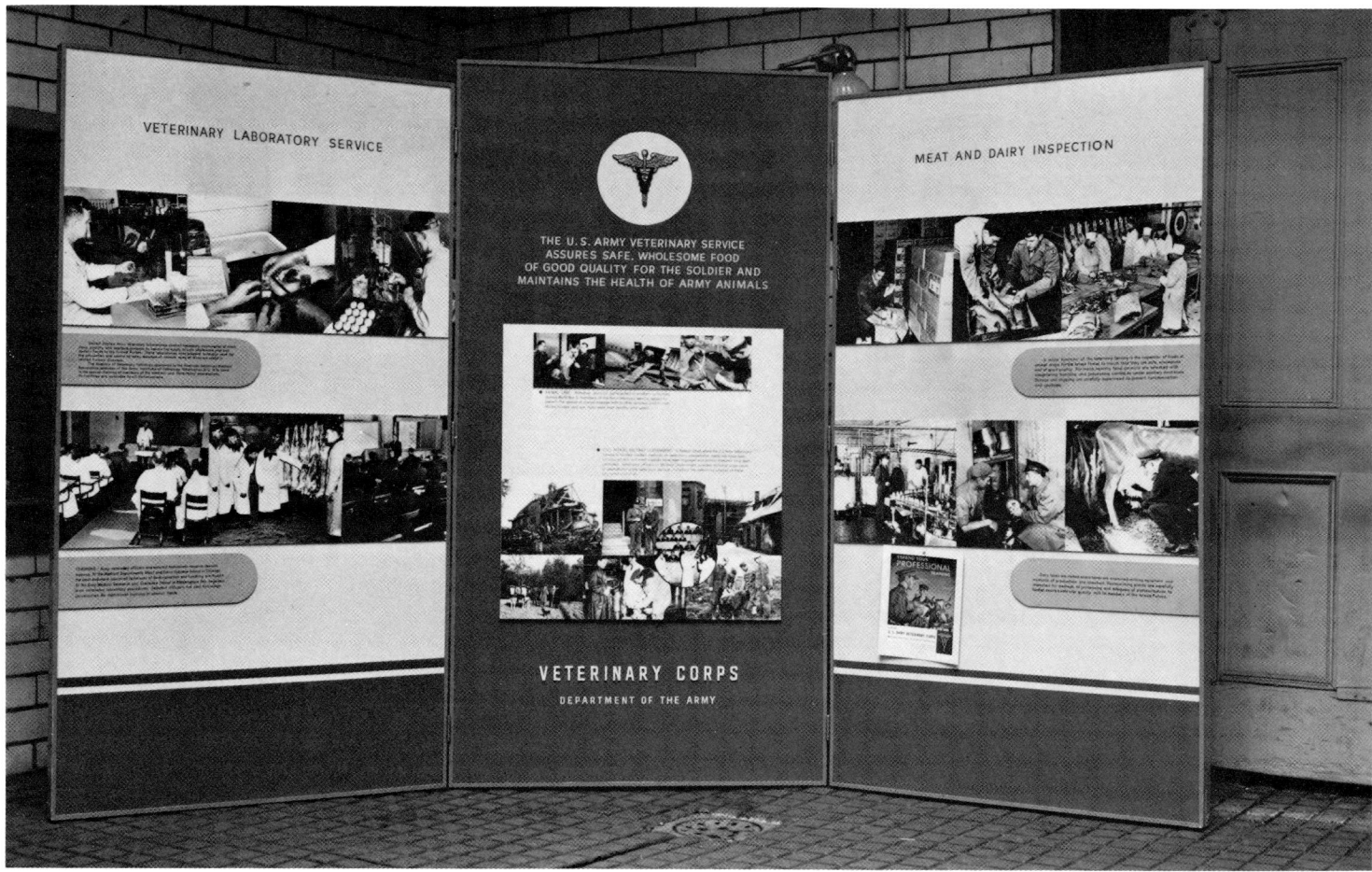

An Army Veterinary Corps display at OSU in 1949. At this point, the position of veterinary medicine in the military services seemed secure. But three decades later Congressional action changed the outlook. (Photo Archives, Ohio State University)

In terms of rank and acceptance, the veterinarian was finally "in the Army now." With America's entry into the First World War, professional veterinary medicine began to assume a significant military role, the importance of which was emphasized by Dr. David S. White, Dean of the OSU Veterinary College. Addressing the 1918 OVMA Annual Meeting, Dean White, then a major in the Army Veterinary Corps, posed a question and provided the answer:

> Why is a veterinary corps needed in the National Army? Even if for the present the Army used no cavalry at the front, there will be employed more animals per man in this war than in any war in history. For each three and a fraction men in the National Army, there is one public animal. If we raise an army of three and a fraction millions of men, one million animals (horses and mules) will be needed.... To (protect the health and preserve the efficiency of these animals), a well-organized, manned and equipped veterinary corps must be available....

Dean White was a leading figure in the Army's veterinary service. While on wartime leave from OSU, he assisted in the organization of the Veterinary Corps and later joined the American Expeditionary Force as Chief Veterinarian. White's contributions led to his promotion to full Colonel; he was the first veterinary officer to hold this rank.

During World War I, a sizable number of Ohio veterinarians entered military service. Their involvement and its home-front impact was noted at the OVMA's 1919 Annual Meeting in remarks by Association President, Dr. A. D. Fitzgerald:

> Approximately 25 percent of the active members of the profession in Ohio heard the call to colors, gave up all private interests, and hastened to meet the emergency that had arisen. (Considering that the veterinary profession) is comprised of approximately 600 duly-qualified men, we can begin to appreciate how severe a drain has been placed upon our manpower. Large areas of this progressive livestock state were left without the services of (these) men.

In recognition of this wartime commitment, the Association had a year earlier passed a resolution stating "that as a tribute to the services of Ohio Veterinarians in the United States Army, the OSVMA obligates itself for membership dues to all members of this association who are commissioned or enlisted in the Army service during the pendency of the war."

World War I confirmed the importance of veterinary service to the military forces. The newly-formed Army Veterinary Corps could not in a single, short conflict, rectify all the mistakes of more than a century, but it made noteworthy progress in raising the standards of military animal care. In the process, it established itself as a viable military unit.

With the outbreak of World War II, veterinary medicine achieved even greater recognition. There were far fewer animals to care for, but this declining responsibility was offset by the need for many other veterinary services. One of the most important of these was noted by Professor Arthur Schalk in his Veterinary College history:

> It can be said that World War II provided an opportunity for the Veterinary Corps of the Army to establish its importance in the war effort through its services in the field of food inspection and supervision. This service was so competently and praiseworthily rendered by the veterinary profession that not a single outbreak of food poisoning occurred during the entire emergency period.... (These) efficient services brought to light quite forcibly the enlarged sphere of importance and usefulness of veterinary medicine in the nation's health and economy.

In addition, military veterinarians also were assigned a wide range of other responsibilities. These included disease control work in war-torn countries and important overseas assignments in the areas of food production, sanitation and animal care.

The expansion and diversification of veterinary medicine during World War II was a major factor in stimulating postwar interest in the veterinary profession. In succeeding years, the responsibilities of military veterinarians continued to increase, with new emphasis on research and veterinary involvement in the emerging field of space medicine. For a brief time, it appeared that veterinary medicine had securely established itself as an essential and progressing military service.

But, ironically, this period proved to be the highwater mark. Expanded responsibilities notwithstanding, there still were people who noted the steady decline of military animal life and questioned the continuing need for veterinarians. In the end their views prevailed and in 1979 Congress ordered a reorganization and reduction of military veterinary services. The action included termination of the Air Force Veterinary Service as of 1980 and the transfer of all veterinary services to the Army. The years since have been marked by a steady decline in the number of military veterinarians and while those remaining still play significant roles, the profession's military visibility is fading.

And what the future holds is still in doubt.

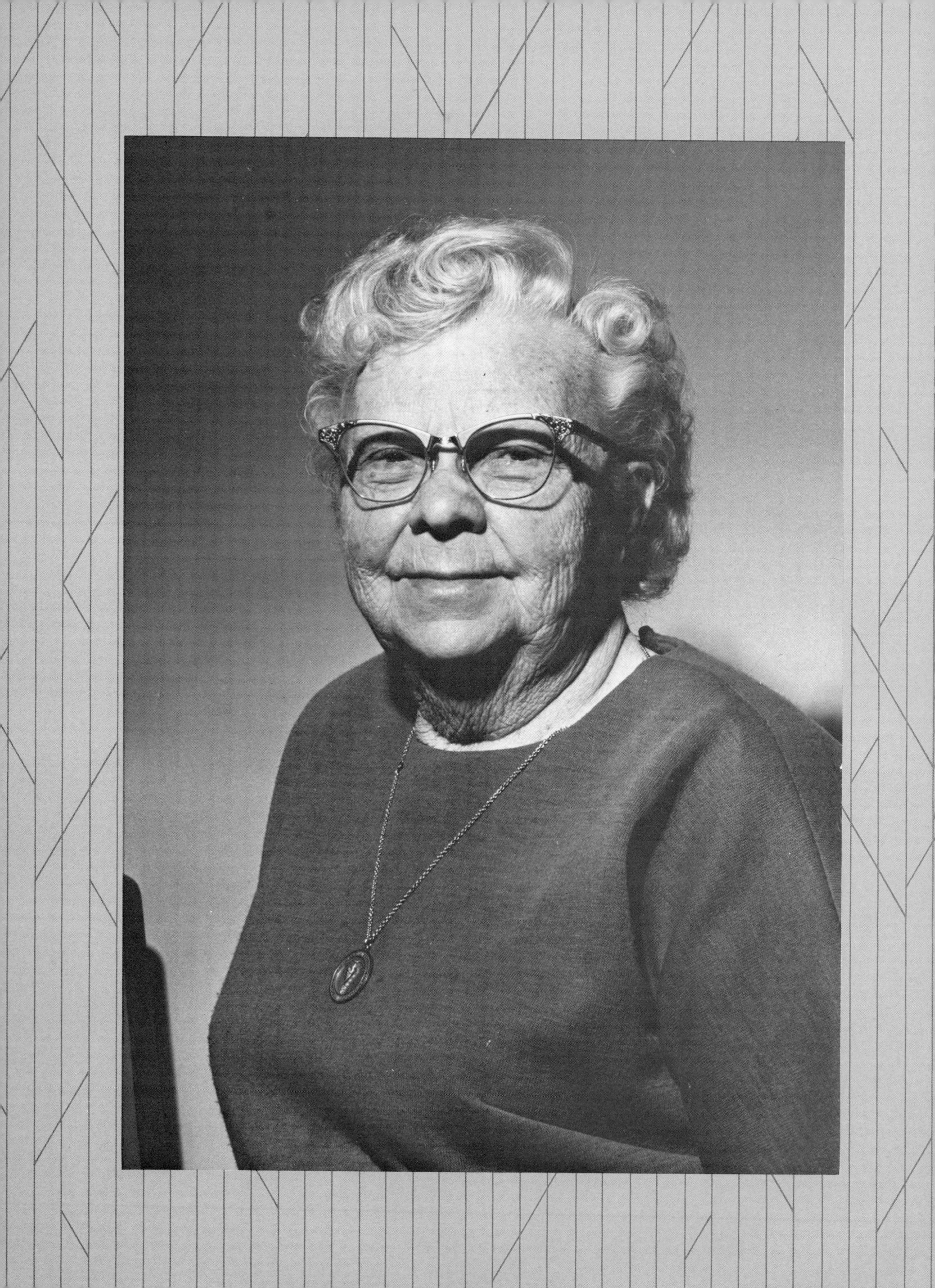

CHAPTER IX

THE OVMA AUXILIARY

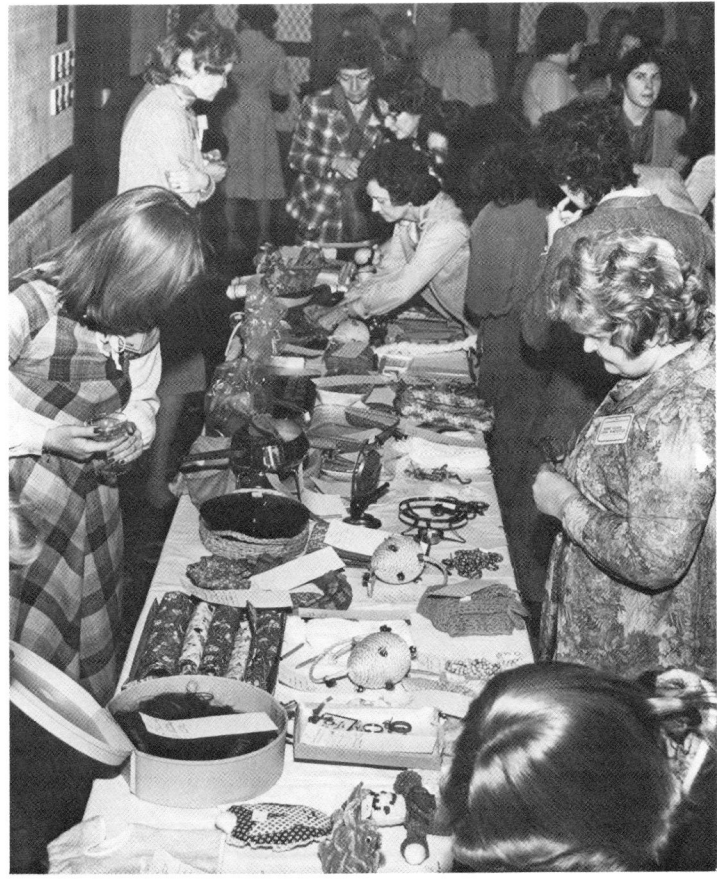

A "Silent Auction," one of the many events initiated by the OVMA Auxiliary to support its public service and education projects. (OVMA Auxiliary files)

In 1939, the OVMA acquired a valuable ally with the formation of the Women's Auxiliary.

Over the years, many of the veterinarians attending Association meetings were accompanied by their wives and as early as 1931 there was an effort to form an auxiliary group. But it was not until 1939 that the goal was realized; that year some 50 women met during the Annual Meeting in Columbus and formed the Women's Auxiliary. The first officers included: President, Mrs. C. H. Case, Akron; Vice President, Mrs. Charles W. Fogle, Leipsic; and Secretary-Treasurer, Mrs. D. M. Swinehart, Elida.

Early on, the new Auxiliary established itself as more than a social group. In 1941, it voted to donate $10.00 to the OSU Veterinary College Library for the purchase of a scientific book and support of the Library fund continued for several years, with contributions being raised to $15.00 in 1942 and $25.00 in 1946. The donations were generous, considering that Auxiliary dues were only 50 cents a year.

In 1944, the Auxiliary adopted a constitution, incorporating three major objectives. They were:

> To assist the profession in informing the public of the value of veterinary service in practice, education, research, public health and sanitation and other fields of endeavor.

> To assist, in some manner, the educational advancement of the students in the College of Veterinary Medicine at Ohio State University.

> To promote good fellowship among the women attending annual meetings of the OVMA.

From this point on, the Auxiliary involved itself in a growing number of projects. One of the most important was initiated in 1961 with the establishment of the "Women's Auxiliary-OVMA Student Loan Fund," designed to aid needy veterinary students at OSU. The first donations included $315.63 from the proceeds of an Auxiliary Christmas card sale and a

Mrs. Lillie Grossman, the "Grand Lady of Veterinary Medicine." (OVMA Auxiliary files)

101

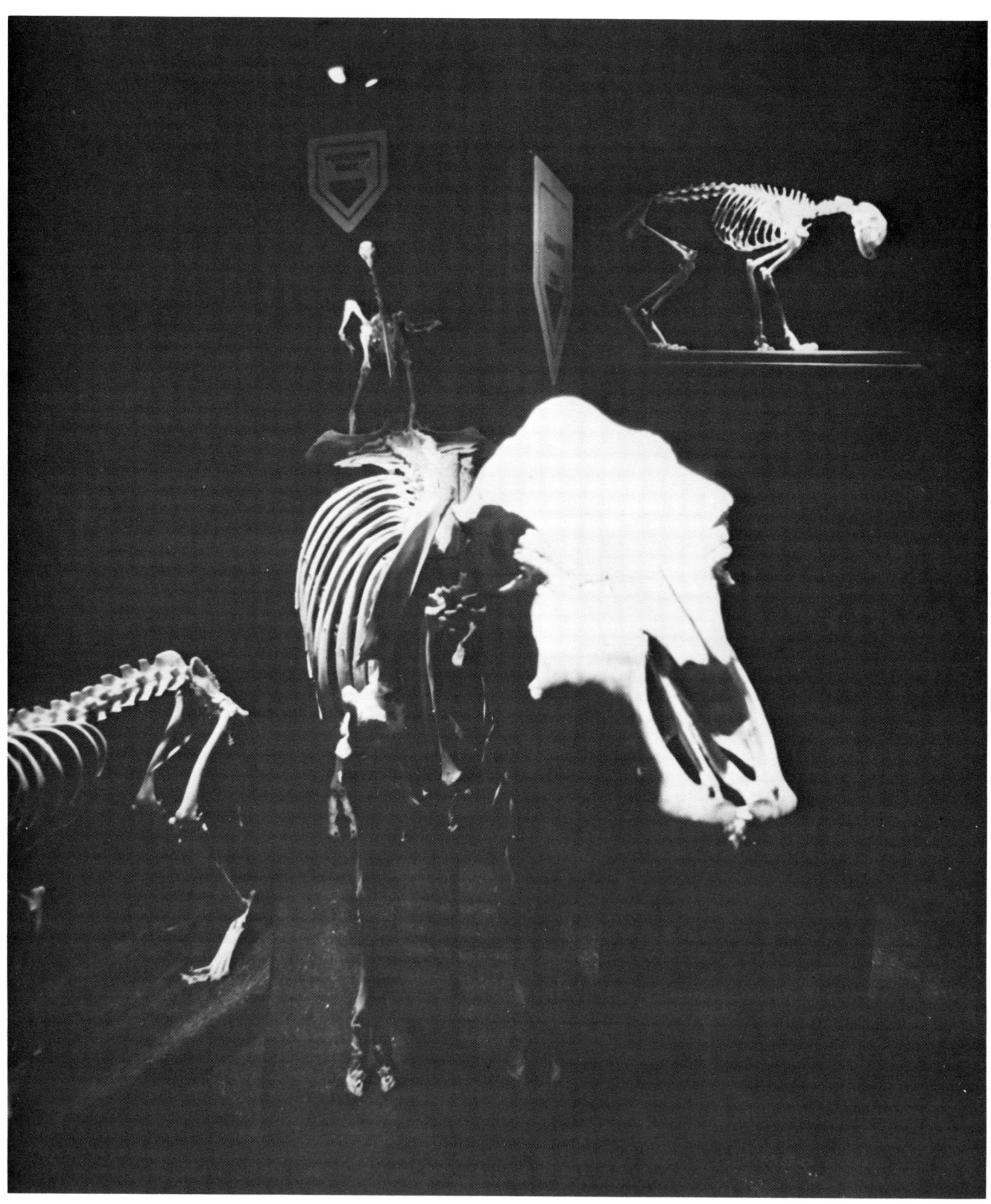

The Veterinary Medicine Exhibit at Columbus' Center of Science and Industry. The Auxiliary played a major role in raising funds for this important display which was dedicated in 1977.

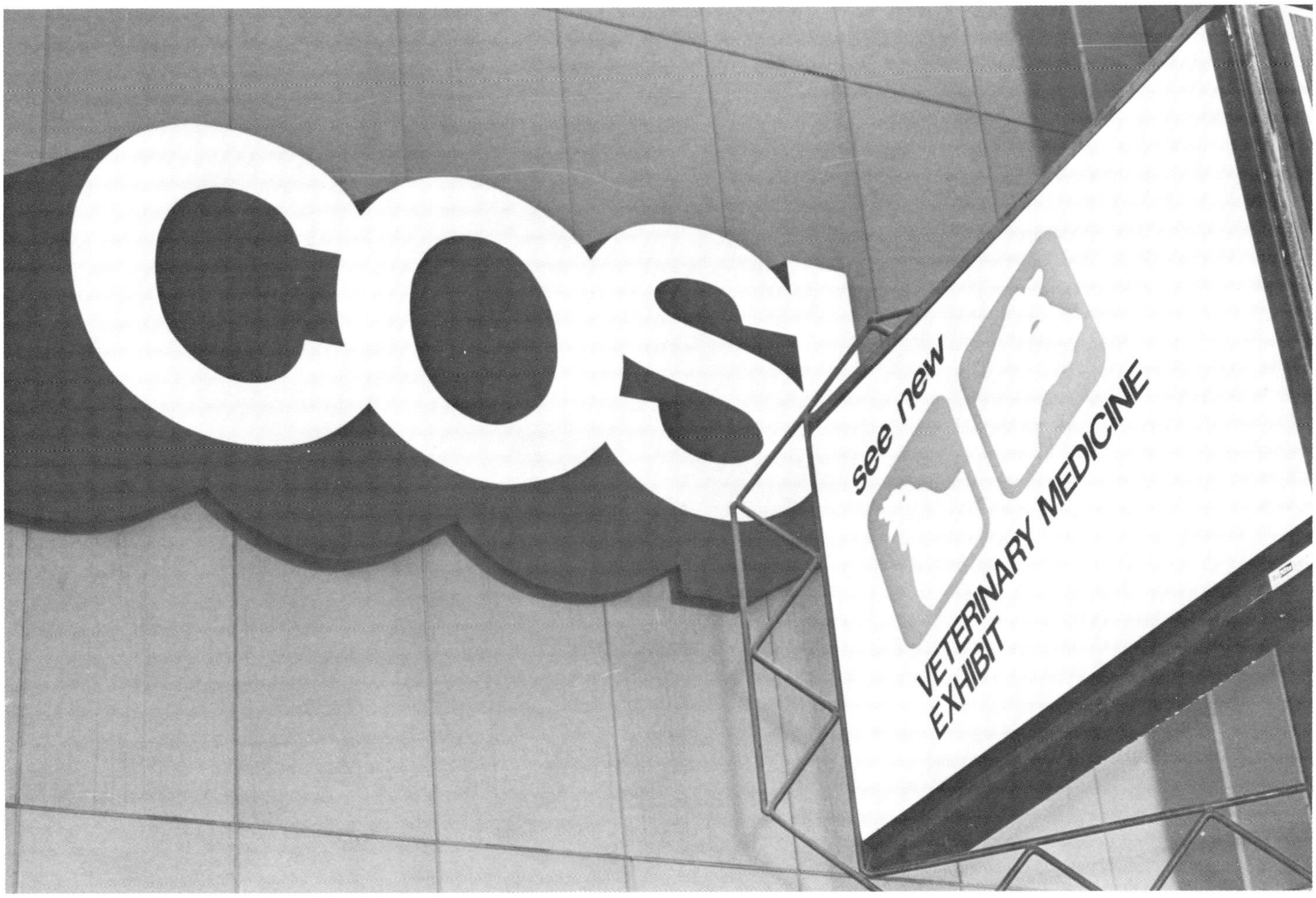

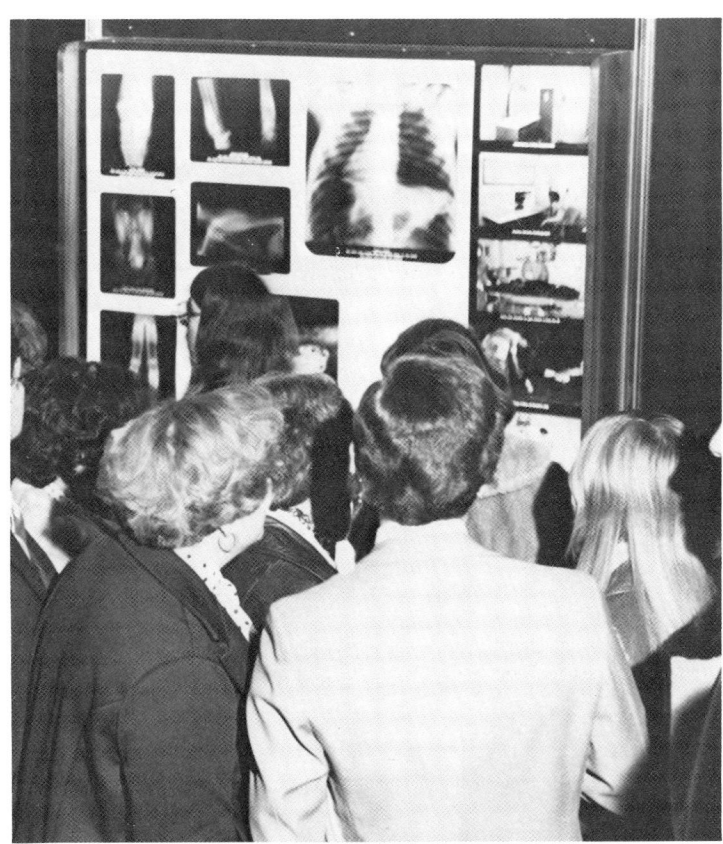
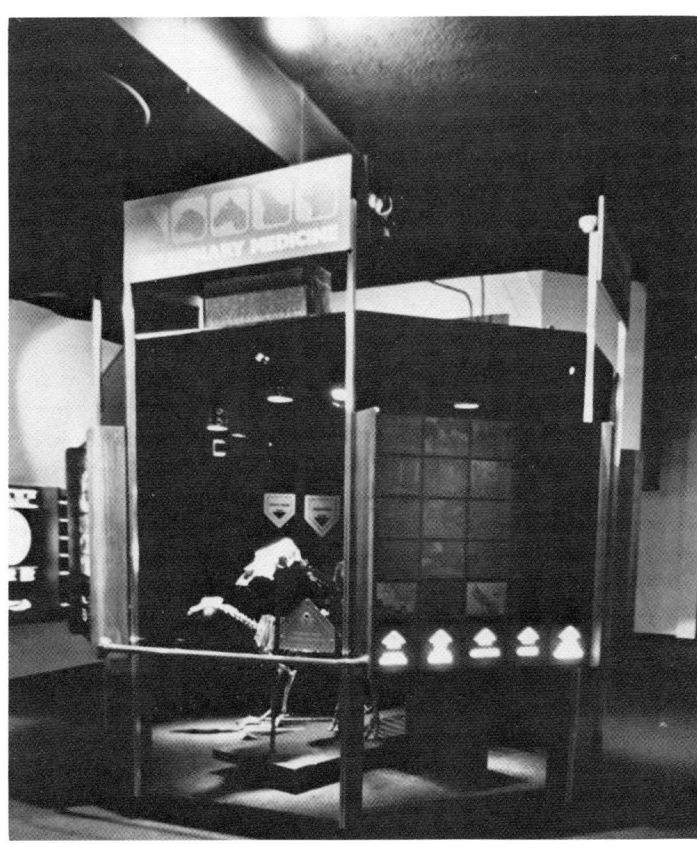

103

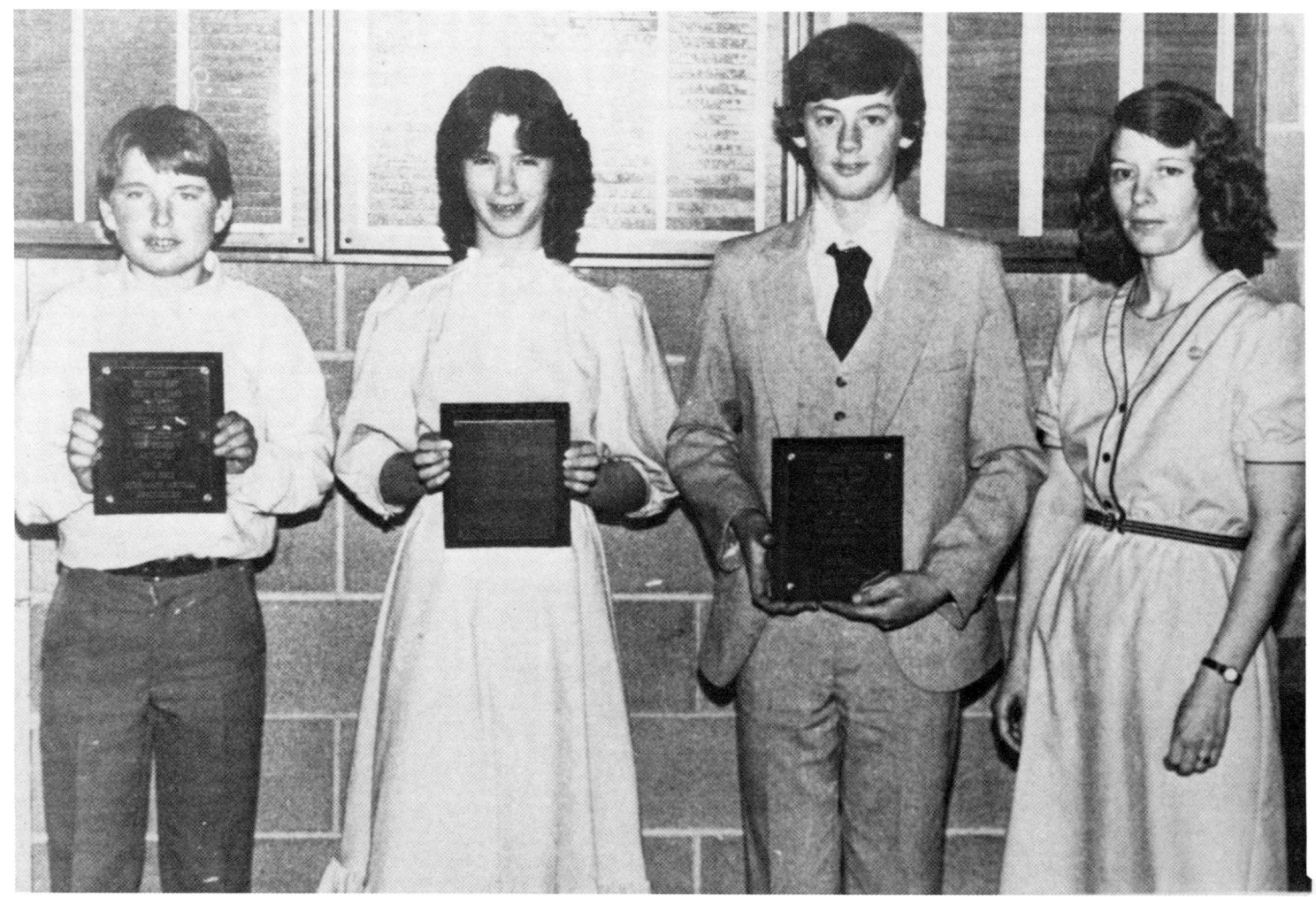

Since 1967 the OVMA Auxiliary has honored the top winners in the state's "Science Day" competition. In 1983 Auxiliary awards went to (left to right) Paul H. Warye, Julie Lashley, and Ronald J. Packard, Jr. With the winning trio is Auxiliary President Mrs. Grant Johnson.

$2,000 contribution from the OVMA. Regulations governing the Fund stipulated that its use be limited to juniors and seniors except in case of extreme emergency. To date, more than 100 Veterinary College students have benefited from the Loan Fund.

Another Auxiliary project involves the presentation of awards to the three top winners in the state's "Science Day" competition. Begun in 1967 as a public relations activity, this is one of the Auxiliary's ongoing projects. Others include support of the AVMA Student Loan Fund, AVMA Research Foundation, AVMA Memorial Fund, Ohio Rural Health Council, Pilot Dogs, Ohio Animal Health Foundation, and the OSU Chapter of the Junior AVMA Auxiliary.

The Auxiliary also has been active in public education efforts. In 1962, it distributed 1,600 "Career Kits" throughout the state and, in 1967, purchased and placed copies of "Veterinarians and What They Do" in all Ohio high school libraries. Other projects have included the distribution in 1978 of the "Animal Studies Resource Booklet" to school libraries throughout the state and the distribution of radio public service announcements and newspaper releases concerning animal health care.

In 1974, the Auxiliary undertook a major effort to help fund an exhibit on Veterinary Medicine at the Center of Science and Industry Museum in Columbus after it was pointed out that the veterinary profession was the only one in the health field without representation at the Center. The fund-raising efforts of the Auxiliary and other groups were successful and the new Veterinary Medicine Exhibit was officially opened on February 7, 1977.

The Auxiliary gained its first male member in 1978; he was Jeff Walton, the husband of Emily Walton who was then a first year student at the OSU Veterinary College. With this gain came a name change; in a 1980 revision of the constitution, the word "Women's" was deleted and the group became the "Auxiliary to the Ohio Veterinary Medical

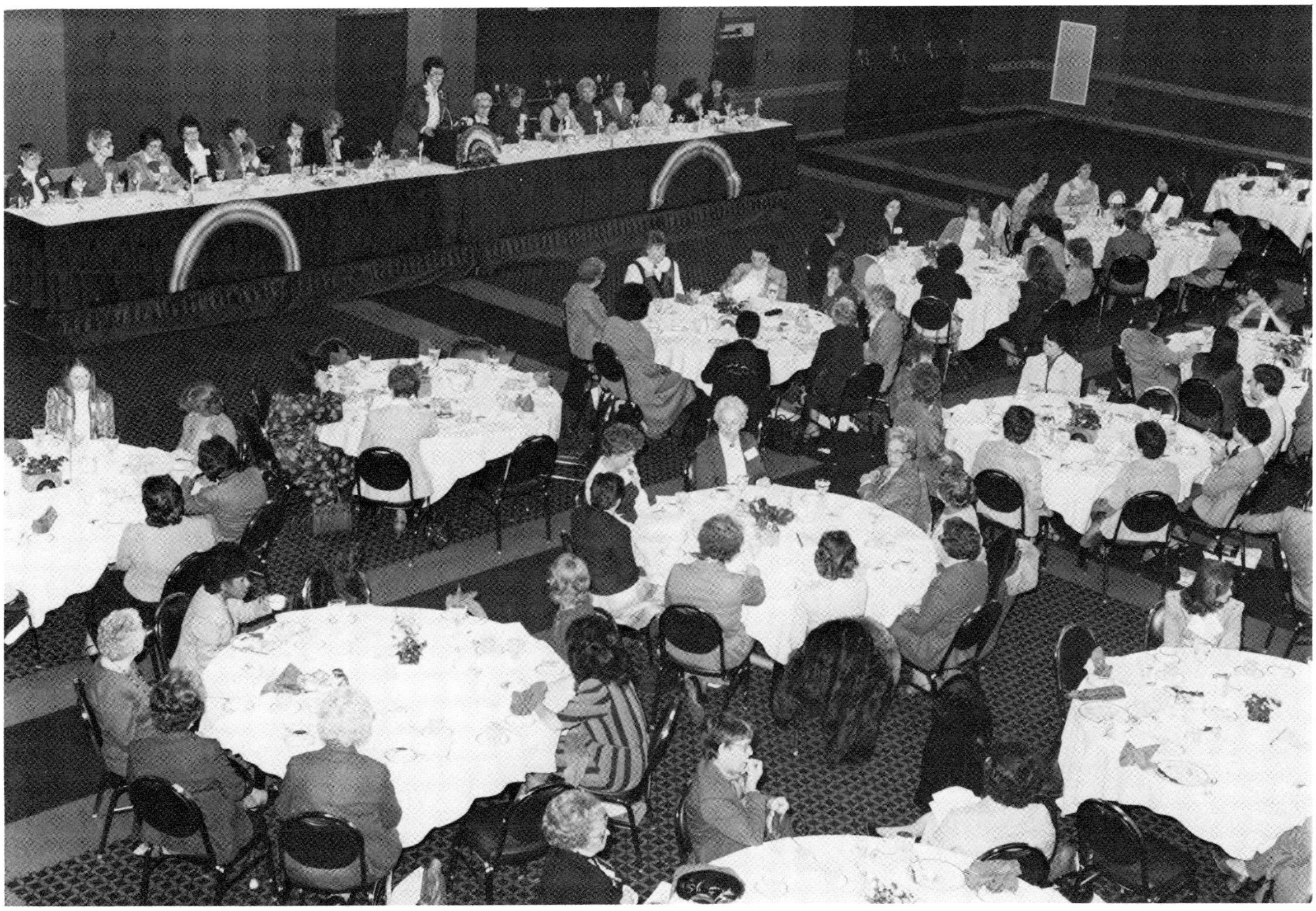

Auxiliary members in session at the 1983 Annual Meeting.

Association." Another constitutional change stipulated that "Membership in the Auxiliary is available to spouses, children, parents, siblings, and widows or widowers of veterinarians who are or were, while still living, in good standing of the Ohio Veterinary Medical Association."

Although the OVMA Auxiliary did not affiliate with the Auxiliary of the AVMA until 1945, two Ohioans already had headed the national group. They were Mrs. Lillie Grossman, a charter member of the national auxiliary, who served as its president from 1930 to 1932, and Mrs. C. H. Case, who was president from 1938 to 1940. Since then, four OVMA Auxiliary members have served as president of the national auxiliary, including Mrs. L. R. Richardson (1954); Mrs. Earl Moore (1955); Mrs. Keith Wearly (1969); and Mrs. David Rickards (1976).

In addition to this recognition, the OVMA Auxiliary has also been the recipient of several awards presented by its national counterpart. Among them are a Certificate of Award given in 1962, Silver Certificates of Achievement on the 1977, 1978, 1980 and 1982 Honor Rolls, and a Maintenance Plus One Certificate presented in 1982.

In 1974, the AVMA Auxiliary paid special tribute to Mrs. Lillie Grossman, the "Grand Lady of Veterinary Medicine" and long-time historian for the OVMA Auxiliary. At the national convention, a resolution was adopted which read:

> In recognition of her faithful and uninterrupted attendance at AVMA conventions during a period which spans fifty-two years, the AVMA Auxiliary does hereby resolve that the Outstanding Senior Wife award silver bowl be known as the Lillie Grossman Bowl.

(The preceding chapter was condensed from the *History of the Auxiliary to the Ohio Veterinary Medical Association* written by Lenna and Dottie Henson in 1983.)

FREE CLINIC HOURS

0130
ANIMAL ROOM
finnigan

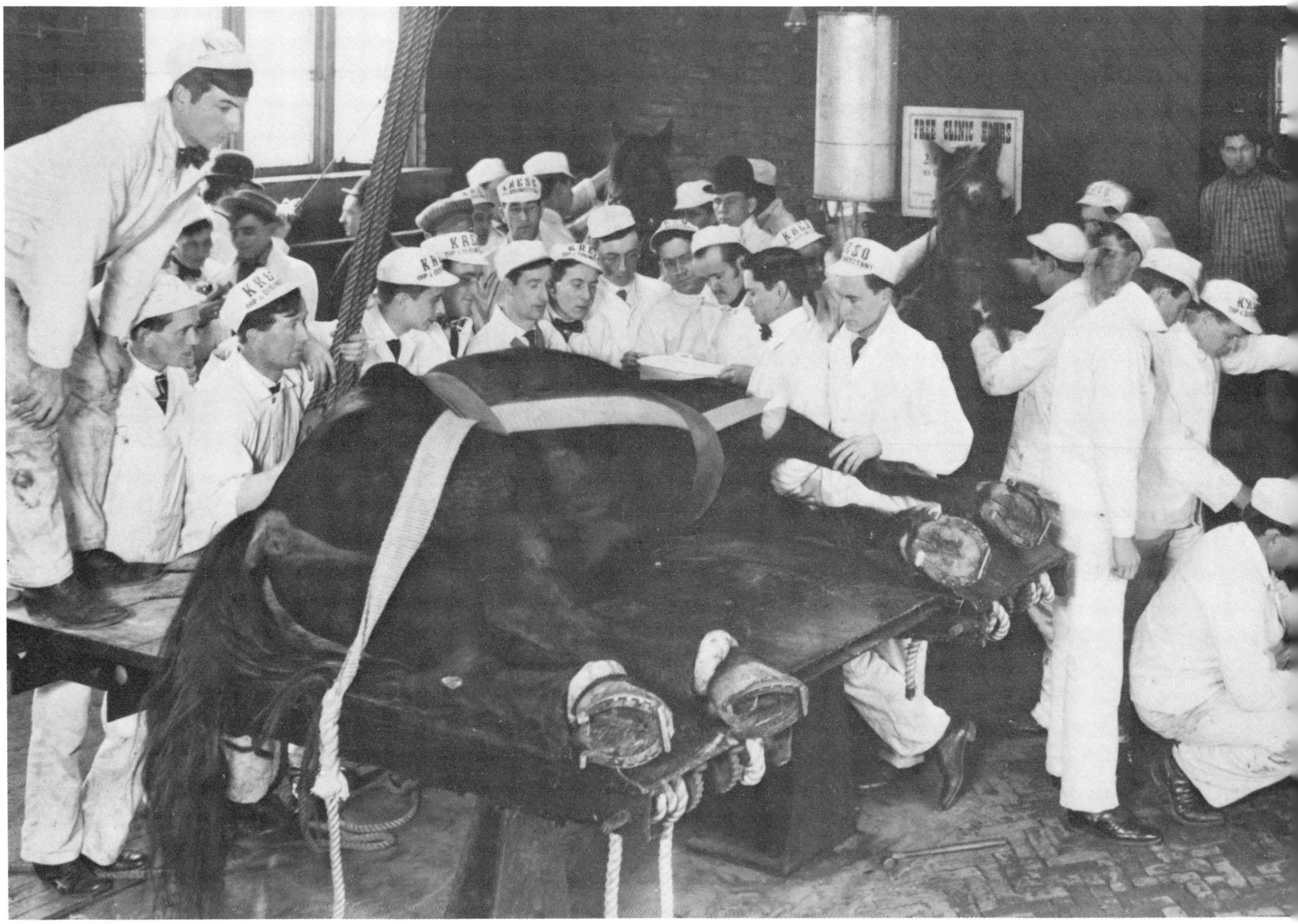

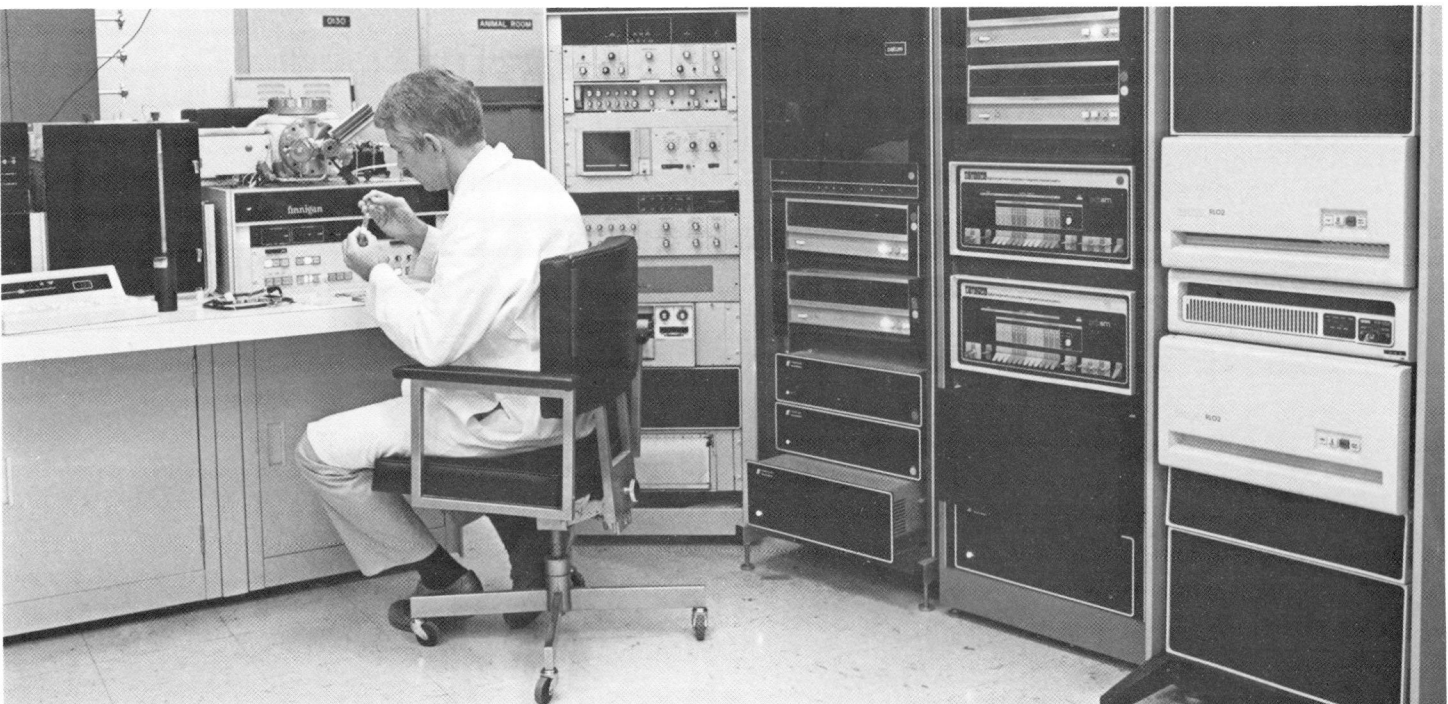

EPILOGUE:
THE FUTURE

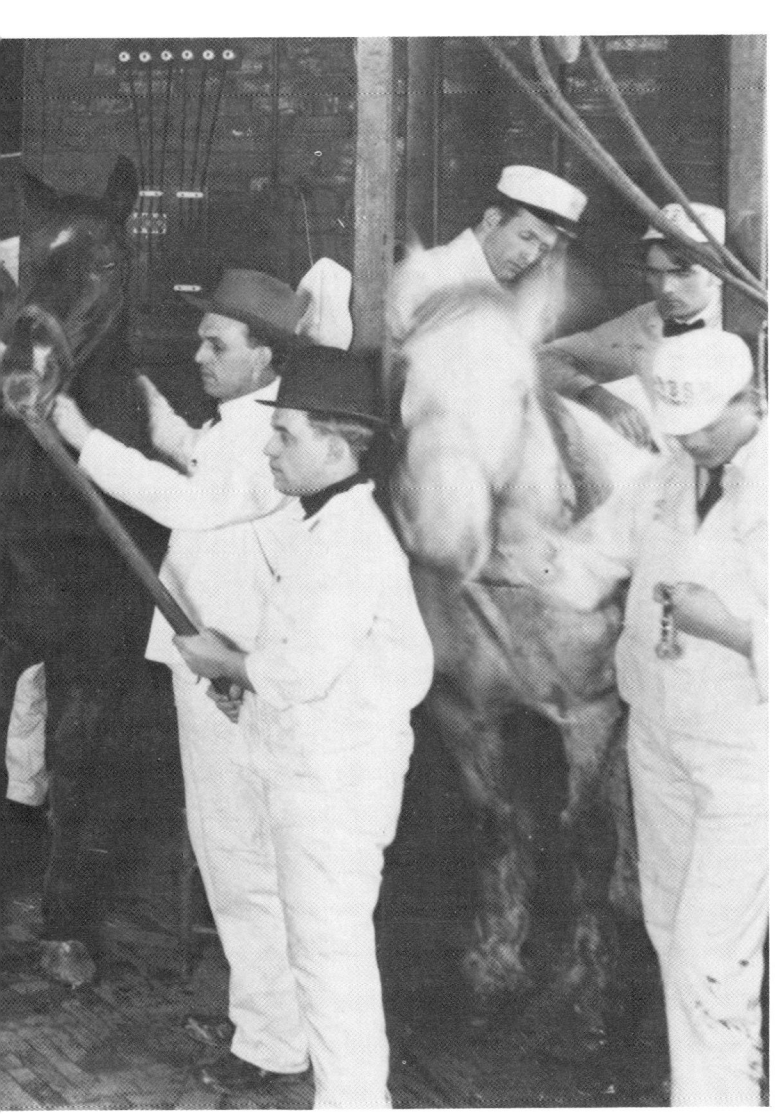

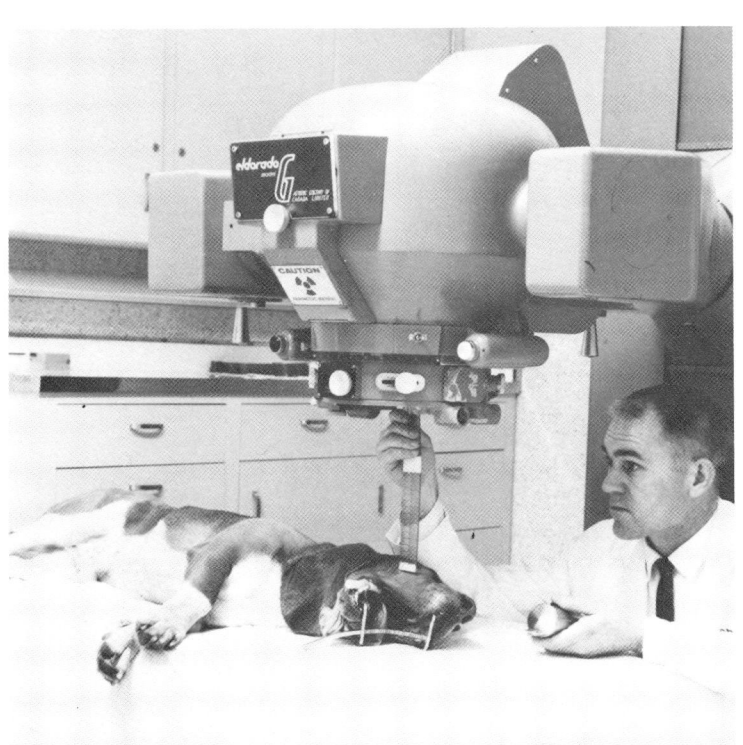

The first Century of Caring is over; the second Century is now in progress. And at this point, no one can forecast with absolute precision the future of veterinary medicine. Perhaps the safest prediction is that it will be marked by the same change and response to change that characterized the past 100 years.

But some things will remain the same. The Veterinarians' Oath speaks of using the skills of the profession "for the benefit of society, through the protection of animal health, the relief of animal suffering, the conservation of livestock resources, the promotion of public health, and the advancement of medical knowledge." This commitment is not going to change; it has guided and shaped the profession throughout its history and it will continue to do so as veterinary medicine enters a future that will be every bit as challenging as the past.

Research is certain to open new fields to veterinarians, as will the growing need for veterinary services, in both emerging and long-established areas of practice. But whatever forms these new responsibilities take, they will be addressed as part of that broader concern for the general welfare of both animals and humans articulated in the Veterinarians' Oath.

Each veterinarian plays a role in translating this oath into practice and so it is individual integrity that counts. Over 75 years ago, Dr. Walter Shaw made a wise observation about this when he addressed the 1916 OVMA Annual Meeting and told colleagues:

> If every member of this profession will conduct himself in a frank and honorable way, and take an active part in the welfare of the community in which he lives, the profession will soon receive the recognition it should have.

The stature of Veterinary Medicine today is conclusive evidence that Dr. Shaw's advice has been heeded. And the words ring as true in 1983 as they did three-quarters of a century ago.

BIBLIOGRAPHY

Yearbooks of the Ohio Veterinary Medical Association, 1911–1952.

The Ohio Veterinarian, OVMA, 1959–1970.

OVMA Newsletter, 1970–1983.

A History of the Veterinary Profession in Ohio, OVMA, 1970.

History of the Auxiliary to the Ohio Veterinary Medical Association, 1983.

History of the College of Veterinary Medicine: OSU 1873–1956, Professor Arthur F. Schalk, Ohio State University Press, 1957.

1970 Centennial History of The College of Veterinary Medicine, Ohio State University.

Speculum, OSU College of Veterinary Medicine, 1977–1981.

Address by Dr. W. Ann Reynolds, Chancellor, The California State University, at the OSU College of Veterinary Medicine, May 13, 1983.

Annual Reports, Ohio State University Research Foundation, 1942–1982.

The Columbus Dispatch, July 25, 1883.

The Ohio Farmer, January 6, 1883; July–October, 1883; January 19 & 26, 1884; October 25, 1884.

The American Veterinary Profession: Its Background and Development, J. F. Smithcors, DVM, PhD., Iowa State University Press, 1963.

A Short History of Veterinary Medicine in America, B. W. Bierer, Michigan State University Press, 1955.

Cattle, Priests and Progress in Medicine, Calvin W. Schwabe, DVM, University of Minnesota Press, 1978.

The Troubled Farmer: 1850–1900, Earl W. Hayter, Northern Illinois University Press, 1968.

Veterinary Medicine and Human Health, Calvin W. Schwabe, DVM, Williams and Wilkins, 1964.

The Ascent of Veterinary Medical Education, Dr. W. W. Armistead, JAVMA, July 1, 1976.

The Growth and Development of Small Animal Practice in the United States, Dr. David M. Drenan, JAVMA, July 1, 1976.

A Brief History of the AVMA. Dr. Arthur Freeman, JAVMA, July 1, 1976.

Ms. Veterinarian, Mary Price Lee, Westminster Press, 1976.

An Exploratory Study of Women in the Health Professions Schools, Volume V: Veterinary Medicine, Department of Health, Education and Welfare, 1976.

First Annual Report, Bureau of Animal Industry, USDA, 1884.

After 1883: One Hundred Years of Organized Veterinary Medicine in Pennsylvania, PVMA, 1982.

PHOTO SOURCES:
Ohio Historical Society
Ohio State University Photo Archives
Ohio State University Press
Photo Files, Ohio Veterinary Medical Association
Photo Files, Auxiliary to the OVMA
Ohio Veterinary Medical Board

The OVMA deeply appreciates the research assistance provided by Ruth Jones, OSU Photo Archives; Arlene Peterson, Ohio Historical Society; Roberta Garrett, OSU College of Veterinary Medicine Library; and Dr. Raimund Coerler, Dr. Robert Bober and Dorothy Ross, OSU Archives.

PAST PRESIDENTS

W. C. Fair*	1883–1885
J. V. Newton	1886
T. B. Cotton	1887
J. C. Meyers, Jr.	1888
J. S. Butler	1889
T. B. Hillock	1890
G. W. Butler	1891
W. R. Howe	1892
W. E. Wight	1893–1894
J. D. Fair	1895–1896
E. H. Shepard	1897–1898
Walter Shaw	1899–1900
S. D. Myers	1901–1902
F. E. Anderson	1903
J. H. Blattenberg	1904
W. E. Clemens	1905
D. S. White	1906
W. A. Axby	1907
C. B. Fredrick	1908
H. Fulstow	1909
W. H. Gribble	1910
L. P. Cook	1911–1912
A. S. Cooley	1913
S. Sisson	1914
F. F. Sheets	1915
Reuben Hilty	1916
Harry T. Moss	1917
A. D. Fitzgerald	1918
W. B. Washburn	1919
O. V. Brumley	1920
C. H. Case	1921
G. W. Cliffe	1922
C. W. Fogle	1923
B. H. Edgington	1924
S. R. Craver	1925
P. T. Engard	1926
J. F. Planz	1927
D. M. Swinehart	1928
F. L. Carr	1929
H. A. Hoopes	1930
F. A. Zimmer	1931
J. N. Shoemaker	1932
O. C. Alspach	1933
E. V. Hover	1934
J. W. Jackman	1935–1936
H. E. Meyers	1937
W. F. Guard	1938
N. D. Backus	1939
H. E. Ash	1940
S. L. Saylor	1941
D. C. Hyde	1942–1943
N. S. Craver	1944
E. M. DeTray	1945
J. H. Lenfestey	1946
A. G. Madden, Jr.	1947
G. W. Lies	1948
R. E. Rebrassier	1949
H. K. Bailey	1950
S. W. Stout	1951
J. T. Burriss	1952
W. O. Keefer	1953
C. W. Cromley	1954
H. B. Roberts	1955
W. H. Pavey	1956
J. L. Boydston	1957
J. A. McCoy	1958
C. D. Barrett	1959
R. L. Rudy	1960
C. S. Alvanos	1961
J. K. Bratton	1962
W. L. Ingalls	1963
W. E. Amling	1964
L. E. Green	1965
J. H. Helwig	1966
D. E. Mossbarger	1967
R. W. Grundish	1968
M. E. Epperson	1969
W. J. Roenigk	1970
M. L. Willen	1971
C. W. Miller	1972
D. M. Drenan	1973
B. S. Henson	1974
G. R. Blind	1975
Vernon Tharp	1976
Dick Johnson	1977
John Moore	1978
Ronald Fuller	1979
Charles Neer	1980
Jack Workman	1981
Milton Wyman	1982
Clyde Purdy	1983

*Historical Note—Some listings of past OVMA presidents inaccurately indicate that Dr. Norton S. Townshend was the first person to hold the association's top office. But as a Medical Doctor, Dr. Townshend was not eligible for the presidency. The position was held by W. C. Fair from the formation of the organization in 1883 until 1885.

WOMEN'S AUXILIARY PRESIDENTS

Mrs. C. W. Case (1st President)	1940
Mrs. C. W. Gogle	1941–1942
Mrs. J. H. Knapp	1943
Mrs. E. V. Hover	1944–1945
Mrs. Earl Starbuck	1947
Mrs. Peter Engard	1948
Mrs. Harold Bond	1949
Mrs. Alan Fogle	1950
Mrs. Vernon Tharp	1951
Mrs. C. J. Griffin	1952
Mrs. Neil Myers	1953
Mrs. Roy Ware	1954
Mrs. Don Mossbarger	1955
Mrs. Paul Soldner	1956
Mrs. L. H. Bremer	1957
Mrs. Curtis Cromley	1958
Mrs. H. T. Deacon	1959
Mrs. H. B. Robert	1960
Mrs. R. J. Custis	1961
Mrs. P. B. Johnston	1962
Mrs. B. S. Henson	1963
Mrs. R. W. Grundish	1964
Mrs. J. E. Fox	1965
Mrs. R. L. McMahan	1966
Mrs. H. F. Bloom	1967
Mrs. Earl Weaver	1968
Mrs. O. W. Fallang	1969
Mrs. D. R. Junk	1970
Mrs. D. A. Rickards	1971
Mrs. Royce Smith	1972
Mrs. M. E. Epperson	1973
Mrs. R. D. Burns	1974
Mrs. R. D. Ramseyer	1975
Mrs. T. W. Gigliotti	1976
Mrs. Donald Noah	1977
Mrs. C. W. Miller	1978
Mrs. John Moore	1979
Mrs. Charles Neer	1980
Mrs. Thomas Henson	1981
Mrs. Lawrence Smith	1982
Mrs. Grant Johnson	1983

INDEX

A Short History of Veterinary Medicine in America, 27
Ackerman, Dr. John, 68
American Animal Hospital Association—AAHA, 63, 64, 65
American Cattle Doctor, 62
American Veterinary Medical Association, 9, 25, 39, 44, 55, 57, 63, 64, 65, 84, 105
Anthrax, 52
Aristotle, 5, 6
Armistead, Dr. W. W., 5
Art of Farriery, 5
Ashcraft, Dr., 68
AVMA Journal, 5

Barrett, Dr. Clinton, 71
Bates, Dr. Morgan, 68
Berry, Dr. V. A., 13
Beutel, Dr. Charles, 18
Bierer, B. W., 27
Billings, Dr. Frank, 65
Boston Veterinary Institute, 9
Bowersmith, Dr. J., 13
Bowler, Dr. George W., 10, 19
Brown, Robert, 84
Brucellosis, 48, 49, 52, 85
Brumley, Dr. O. V., 25, 63
Burris, Dr. James T., 81
Butler, Dr. J. C., 13

Camper, Dr. Peter, 7
Case, Dr. Claude, 45, 84
Case, Mrs. C. H., 101, 105
Cincinnati Veterinary College, 28, 57
Cliffe, Dr. G. W., 44
Cobalt Therapy, 85
Columbus Dispatch, 14, 15
Cook, Dr. L. P., 23
COSI, 102, 103, 104
Cotton, Dr. T. B., 13, 18, 19
Cunningham, Dr. A. E., 62

Daniels, T. E., 13, 14
Deaton, Dr. Van S., 22, 23
Derr, Dr. W. F., 19
Detmers, Dr. H. J., 22, 28, 34, 35, 37, 38, 39, 52, 85
Diseases of the Small Domestic Animals, 63
Dodd, Dr. George, 62
Dodge, Dr. Ida Mae, 93
Drenan, Dr. David, 62, 64

Edgington, Dr., 49
Epizootic Disease, 2, 4, 6, 43, 55, 65, 73

Fair, Dr. W. C., 18, 19
Fitts, Dr. Robertta Laughlin, 94
Fitzgerald, Dr. A. D., 98
Flynn, Dr. J. C., 65
Fogle, Mrs. Charles W., 101
Foot Rot in Sheep, 1
Foot-and-Mouth Disease, 43, 44, 52, 60
Francis, Dr. Mark, 49, 52, 53

Galen, 5, 6
Geyer, Dr., 49
Glanders of Horses, 1
Gorman Hip Joint, 85, 86
Gorman, Dr. Harry, 85, 86
Great Depression, 61, 81
Greenlee, Dr., 49
Gribble, Dr. William H., 14
Grossman, Lillian, 101, 105

Hawkins, Dr., 18
Hayes, Woody, 75
Hayter, Earl W., 2, 7, 9

Hillock, Dr. T. B., 13, 19
Hilty, Dr. Reuben, 25, 45
Hippocrates, 5
History of the College of Veterinary Medicine, 32
Hog Cholera, 1, 33, 38, 43, 47, 48, 52, 60, 85
Howe, Dr., 18

Jackman, Dr. John, 48, 49
Johnson, Dr. J. W., 62
Johnson, Mrs. Grant, 104
Jones, Dr. W. G., 13

Karb, George J., 55
Kimball, Dr. Florence, 93
King, Gene P., 79
Krill, Dr. Walter R., 75, 76, 81
Labron, Dr. W. A., 13
Lambert F. A., 13
Lampas (disease), 4
Liautard, Dr. Alexandre, 44

Marlin, Dr. T. G., 13, 18
McClaskey, Dr. Walter, 77
McLean, Dr. Lachlan, 44
Moore, Mrs. Earl, 105
Morr, Dr. A., 13
Morrill Act, 10, 28

New York College of Veterinary Surgeons, 9
Newton, Dr. J. V., 13, 14, 15, 18, 19
Nicholson, Dr. Mignon, 93

Ohio Agricultural and Mechanical College—See OSU, 2, 27, 28
Ohio Agricultural Experiment Station, 38, 39
Ohio Agriculture College, 27
Ohio Animal Health Foundation, 73
Ohio Department of Agriculture, 28
    Division of Animal Industry, 66
Ohio Department of Health, 68
Ohio Legislature, 21, 25
    Legislation: Veterinary Practice Act, 20, 25
            H.B. 335, 22
            H.B. 429, 25
Ohio Public Health Federation, 65
Ohio State Board of Veterinary Examiners, 79
Ohio State Fair, 14, 84, 87
Ohio State Journal, 68
Ohio State University, 13, 15, 27, 28, 29, 38, 39, 60, 61, 63, 68, 71, 85, 98
    College of Veterinary Medicine, 2, 15, 22, 31, 32, 35, 39, 41, 43, 49, 52, 60, 63, 64, 71, 72, 75, 81, 85, 91, 93, 94, 95, 98, 101
    Isolation Ward, 35, 41
    Leonard W. Goss Laboratory, 82, 83
    School of Veterinary Medicine, 34
    Sisson Hall, 83
    Veterinary Clinic, 32, 33, 35, 41, 62, 64, 83
    Veterinary Hospital, 31, 35
    Veterinary Laboratory, 32
Ohio State Veterinary Medical Association—See OVMA, 14, 18, 19, 22, 52, 68, 99
Ohio Veterinary Medical Association, 9, 10, 13, 14, 15, 18, 19, 20, 21, 22, 23, 25, 33, 38, 39, 43, 44, 45, 53, 55, 60, 62, 64, 65, 72, 73, 76, 77, 79, 83, 84, 94, 97, 101, 104, 107
    Annual Meeting, 13, 18, 19, 21, 22, 23, 25, 39, 44, 45, 46, 47, 48, 55, 60, 62, 64, 65, 68, 71, 75, 79, 81, 97, 98, 101, 105, 107
    Committee on Diseases, 47
    Legislative Committee, 39, 46
    Progress and Education Committee, 47, 60, 97
    Public Health Committee, 49, 68
Ohio Veterinary Medical Association Auxiliary, 101, 102, 104, 105
Ohio Veterinary Medical Board, 25, 77

Planz, Dr. John F., 68, 84
Pleuropneumonia or Pneumonia, 1
Public Health, 71, 72

Quackery (quacks), 3, 4, 7, 10, 20, 21, 22, 23, 25
Rabies, 71, 72
Rebrassier, Dr. R. E., 25
Reynolds, Dr. W. Ann, 85, 86
Reynoldsberg Diagnostic Laboratory, 66
Richardson, Mrs. L. R., 105
Rickards, Mrs. David, 105
Rinderpest, 6, 7
Rose, Dr. J., 13
Roshon, Charles O., 25

Salihotra, 5
Salmon, Dr. D. E., 52
Scabies, 52
Schalk, Dr. Arthur F., 2, 5, 6, 32, 34, 35, 38, 57, 60, 61, 71, 99
Schwabe, Dr. Calvin, 65
Scothorn, Dr. Ray, 32
Scott, Dr. William, 28, 34
Shaw, Dr. Walter, 13, 19, 21, 107
Sisson, Dr. Septimus, 3, 36, 43, 44, 83
Smith, Dr. Mervin G., 75
Smith Dr. Nathaniel B., 24, 25
Smithcors, J. F., 43, 44, 52
Stange, Dr. C. H., 55
Swine Plague, 1, 38
Swinehart, Mrs. D. M., 101

Texas Cattle Fever, 1, 43, 49, 52
Tharp, Dr. Vernon, 25
The American Veterinary Journal, 1, 5, 62
The American Veterinary Profession, 43
The Anatomy of Domestic Animals, 3, 36
The Ascent of Veterinary Medical Education, 5
The Dog, 62
The First Hundred Years: A Family Album of the Ohio State University, 1870–1970, 37, 41
The Growth and Development of Small Animal Care, 62
The Ohio Farmer, 10, 15, 18, 19, 34, 44, 45, 46, 47, 48
The Ohio Veterinarian, 73, 75
The Troubled Farmer, 2, 7
The United States Farriery, 3, 8
Theobald, Dr. Arthur C., 64
Thompson, Dr. W. O., 52
Townshend, Dr. N. S., 13, 14, 15, 18, 28, 32, 33, 34, 39, 85
Tuberculosis of Cattle, 1, 19, 44, 45, 46, 52
Tuberculosis/Bovine Tuberculosis, 19, 43, 44, 45, 46, 47, 48, 49, 52, 68, 85
Tuttle, Dr. Albert A., 28, 29, 33, 39, 41

United States Air Force, 99
United States Army, 97, 99
United States Bureau of Animal Industry, 57
United States Department of Agriculture, 4, 7, 35, 65
United States Veterinary Medical Association—See AVMA, 9, 10, 25

Vegetius Renatus, 5, 6
Veterinarians and What They Do, 104
Veterinary College of Philadelphia, 9
Veterinary Papyrus of Kahun, 4
Veterinary Practice Act (Practice Act), 20, 22, 23, 25, 76, 77, 79
Voith, Dr. Victoria, 86

Waddel, Dr. J. S., 13
Walton, Dr. Emily, 104
Walton, Jeff, 104
Wearly, Mrs. Keith, 105
Wenger, Dr. Bruce, 68, 84
White, Dr. David S., 25, 37, 98
Whitehead, Dr. 19
Wight, Dr. W. E., 13
Wilson, Dr. Judson W., 86
Women in Veterinary Medicine, 93

Youatt, William, 62

Zimmer, Dr. Fred A., 25, 46, 48